TALES F
KENTUCKY NURSES

TALES FROM
KENTUCKY
NURSES

William Lynwood Montell

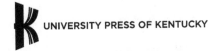

UNIVERSITY PRESS OF KENTUCKY

Scholarly publisher for the Commonwealth,
serving Bellarmine University, Berea College, Centre College
of Kentucky, Eastern Kentucky University, The Filson Historical Society,
Georgetown College, Kentucky Historical Society, Kentucky State University,
Morehead State University, Murray State University, Northern Kentucky University,
Transylvania University, University of Kentucky, University of Louisville, and
Western Kentucky University.
All rights reserved.

Editorial and Sales Offices: The University Press of Kentucky
663 South Limestone Street, Lexington, Kentucky 40508-4008
www.kentuckypress.com

The Library of Congress has cataloged the hardcover edition as follows:

Montell, William Lynwood, 1931-
  Tales from Kentucky nurses / William Lynwood Montell.
    pages cm
  ISBN 978-0-8131-6071-9 (hardcover : acid-free paper) —
  ISBN 978-0-8131-6073-3 (PDF) — ISBN 978-0-8131-6072-6 (ePub)
  1. Nursing—Kentucky—History—Anecdotes. 2. Nurses—Kentucky—
Biography—Anecdotes. I. Title.
  RT5.K46M66 2015
  610.73092'2769—dc23

                    2014044817

ISBN 978-0-8131-6825-8 (pbk. : alk. paper)

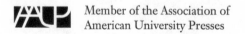

CONTENTS

Introduction

As I have said numerous times to people who come to hear my stories and viewpoints about various topics, I am not interested in writing books about kings, queens, and presidents; my desire is to write about local life and culture relative to professional groups and subregional areas. Thus my professional desire is to help preserve the legacy of local history, life, and culture. To do this, I interview local individuals who can tell their favorite stories about themselves and their work, ranging from humorous to very serious events, or about others in the same profession who serve in various counties across the Commonwealth. Their stories may also be about colleagues now deceased.

My interest in obtaining stories from Kentucky nurses resulted from my work on a number of books published by the University Press of Kentucky, including *Tales from Kentucky Lawyers* (2003), *Tales from Kentucky Doctors* (2008), *Tales from Kentucky Funeral Homes* (2009), *Tales from Kentucky One-Room School Teachers* (2011), and *Tales from Kentucky Sheriffs* (2011). Since all of these books focused on significant professional groups that truly serve Kentucky statewide or in subregional areas, I felt it was high time to obtain stories from nurses. Readers of this book will come away with a full understanding of the importance of nurses and why doctors, hospitals, and local residents could not do without their services. I offer my thanks for the services and devoted thoughts of nurses and all others whose desire is to help fulfill the informational needs of everyone in the wonderful state of Kentucky.

The bulk of the stories in this book are about nurses during their active years, and most are about their professional practices. Just like physicians, these nurses encountered various forms of sickness, sadness, humorous occurrences, and death, which in some instances brought tears to the eyes of nurses who had strived to help their patients through long periods of sickness. Whether humorous or sad, stories such as these are historically important as a means of preserving valid information about the life and times of twentieth- and twenty-first-century nurses.

The stories range from the very brief to the lengthy, with many in between. The majority provide information about events that occurred within the past twenty to thirty years, but some reach back to the 1920s and 1930s.

The nurses who provided these stories are professionally licensed individuals. Although a few of those who shared stories with me are relatively young, I typically contacted middle-age or older nurses, as they were likely to have memorable accounts of professional nursing services that would help readers understand how healing work-services used to be. They willingly shared their professional memories, and virtually all of them sent their stories and viewpoints to me via e-mail. Very few were verbally tape-recorded or handwritten and mailed to me. Patients' names are not revealed in order to protect their privacy.

The nurses and former nurses included in this book, and the area where each worked, are as follows: Evelyn Pearl Anderson (London), Teresa Bell (Wingfield, Edmonson County), Mary Lewis Biggerstaff (Frontier Nursing Service [FNS], Berea), Helen E. Browne (FNS), Jana Buckles (Lawrenceburg), Dana Burnam (Bowling Green), Jenny Burton (Bowling Green), Ruth A. Buzzard (Dawson Springs), Dorothy Caldwell (FNS, Burlington), Rebecca Collins (Auburn), Jean Fee (FNS), Terry Foody (Oldham County), Carolyn Booth Gregory (FNS), Mary Hawkes (FNS), Martha Hill (Glendale), Fredericka Holdship (FNS), Gertrude Isaacs (FNS), Theresa Sue Milburn King (Danville), Mary Lansing (FNS), Georgia Ledford (FNS), Molly Lee (FNS), Betty Lester (FNS), Agnes Lewis (FNS), Elsie Maier (FNS), Marilyn Kaye Montell (Louisville), Chesa Montgomery (Bowling Green), Carrie M. Parker (FNS), Mary Penton (FNS), Nancy N. Porter (FNS), Grace Reeder (FNS), Bobbi Dawn Rightmyer (Harrodsburg), Kay T. Roberts (Jefferson County), Karen Slabaugh (FNS), Patricia A. Slater (Petersburg), Clara Fay Smith (Erlanger), Janet Smith (Irvine), Lydia Thompson (FNS), Jean Tolk (FNS), Charlene Vaught (Portland, TN), Louise Webb (Bowling Green), Martha Webster (FNS), Jo Ann M. Wever (Springfield), Jeri R. White (Lexington), George W. Williams (London), Anne Winslow (FNS), Mary Wiss (FNS, Pike County).

The stories are organized into chapters by subject. "The Frontier Nursing Service" describes the origins and development of that organization, the difficulties that nurses, doctors, and local individuals faced in traveling to a secluded patient's home, and the procedures they followed when they provided medical care. "Emergency Room Episodes" is filled with all variety of dangerous events. "Baby Births" recounts inspirational, even surprising, events that may remind readers of births in their families or communities. "Humorous Accounts" are varied in content and will surprise and thrill readers in various ways. "Patient Misbehavior" describes activities that range from serious to unforgettable to humorous. "Inspirational Tales" shows the heart-filled devotion that nurses bring to their services to patients. In "Nursing Training and Career Memories," storytellers describe why they decided to become nurses, the types of schools they attended, and their services to both adults and children. "Doctors and Nurse Interns" is brief, but it provides important information about medical providers who are still in the early learning stages of their careers. "Various Types of Stories" primarily describes early nursing years relative to things such as thievery and family monetary needs, along with how some nurses tried to help those in need. "Governmental and Business Issues" considers Medicare and Medicaid, along with numerous other concerns relative to monetary needs. "Medications in Earlier Times" gathers stories related to pioneer times and the Frontier Nursing Service up to the 1960s, as well as discussing folk remedies utilized by residents in secluded country areas where doctors and nurses were seldom, if ever, requested.

The reason so many of the stories in this book focus on Leslie County is because that area is the site of rich historical information about the Frontier Nursing Service. Founded by Mary Breckinridge in Hyden, Leslie County, in 1925, the FNS was the leading factor in the provision of health services to people in remote and underserved areas around Hyden. In order to reach distant patients, nurses either walked or rode horses during the early years, but they were provided with jeeps once such vehicles became available. Stories about the Frontier Nursing Service vividly describe nurses, midwives, couriers, and doctors and the services they rendered. Without the assistance of the Louie B. Nunn Center for Oral History, University of Kentucky Libraries, Lexington, interviews with former members of the FNS would likely have never been gathered.

Like my other books about various professional groups, the present book will be appreciated by historians, educators, medical professionals, and residents across the state of Kentucky. I hope that these stories will encourage other types of professionals to consider working on a book featuring their own professions. All of their descriptive stories would provide an important insight into Kentucky's cultural legacy.

I truly have a deep appreciation for all the nurses who took time to share their memories for inclusion in this book. Nurses made and continue to make fabulous contributions to our daily livelihood. Their stories complement formal historical sources. Together, these two types of sources will forever let progenitors know what life and times were like during the eras covered herein. Present nurses whose memorable stories are not included need to personally and regularly write down descriptions of the spectacular services they render, so that their grandchildren and great-grandchildren, as well as future nurses, can learn what work was like for them.

In the words of Evelyn Pearl Anderson, a resident of London, Kentucky, "Nursing is a wonderful profession and for me it was a calling. Nursing goes beyond the shots and bedpan image; it is one to one with needful persons. Nursing does not have to take place in a hospital or doctor's office. It can be in a classroom, on a battlefield, and also in a rural or urban house. Nursing is a 'ministry of the heart.'"[1]

Note

1. Evelyn Pearl Anderson, London, Kentucky, July 18, 2012.

THE FRONTIER NURSING SERVICE

The Frontier Nursing Service was founded in 1925 by Mary Breckinridge in Hyden, a small town in Leslie County, Kentucky. As the director of the FNS for forty years, Mrs. Breckinridge traveled around to mountain counties in the area, talking to judges, doctors, local midwives, and others, asking them to provide various types of services to family and community members who needed help. Mrs. Breckinridge was also responsible for service outposts at Beech Fork, Confluence, Red Bird, Flat Creek, Burlington, Burgess, and Wendover.

The stories in this chapter provide information about services performed by FNS nurses, nurse-midwives, and couriers. Couriers were not nurses, but they assisted FNS nurses in any way possible. They acted as escorts for visitors, treated sick and crippled horses, and rode horses to receive and deliver messages, including postal service mail. FNS staff not only assisted people who were sick but also helped them obtain food, clothing, and other daily necessities and saw to it that children were able to attend school, which could involve a long walk or horse ride to get there. Many stories also tell about early nurses who likewise rode horses or walked along secluded walking trails to reach the homes of their patients.

FRONTIER NURSING SERVICE ORIGINS

It was May 28, 1925, when the lobby of the little Capital Hotel in Frankfort, Kentucky, was buzzing with activity. Not even during a session of the General Assembly of the commonwealth were there more people going and coming. The hotel was the scene of a meeting called by Mrs. Mary Breckinridge for the purpose of founding the Kentucky Committee for Mothers and Children.

The meeting was under way behind closed doors in the assembly room of the hotel. At Mrs. Breckinridge's request Judge Edward O'Rear, a well-known Kentucky jurist who had opened the meeting, briefly stated its purpose to the audience, which included many prominent Kentuckians (and a number of Mary's relatives) and called for an election of officers.

Mary's eyes danced as she looked about her and reflected that more than half the people present were related to her by bloodlines or marriage. . . . In his opening remarks Judge O'Rear prophesied success for the program because of its "sublime audacity." He said that he knew the mountains, because as a young man he had lived in them. His forebears had been a part of them. He liked to think that what the mountain people had to offer was a part of the heritage of America. "Wherever you find a highland people, they are the seed corn of the world," he said in conclusion.

Mary Breckinridge nodded in confirmation. She felt she had come to know the mountain people, and no one was more aware than she of their solid worth and moral integrity. . . . "I can tell you very little you do not already know," she began. "I have been telling the same story over and over ever since I returned from France. I have been telling it with increasing frequency since the summer I spent in the mountains of Kentucky. It was during those months that I made up my mind to spend the rest of my life there in alleviating the unspeakable conditions which have arisen there. . . .

"Friends, you need not imagine such a region. It is there in Leslie County, Knott County, and Owsley County, where I propose with your help to carry on a nursing-midwife service. It will have a double purpose. It will save lives in the mountains of Kentucky. If it is successful, and I promise you it will be, it will be a beacon to the forgotten frontiers not only in our own United States but all over the world. Frankly, I expect nurse volunteers to come to us from the far corners of the earth."

On August 22, 1925, the Leslie County Committee held its initial meeting. . . . An air of excitement pervaded the little mountain town of Hyden. . . . The nursing-midwives and the mountain people who knew Mary Breckinridge had already given her their hearts and trust. . . .

Every citizen of Hyden was well aware that big things were under way. They were proud of their town, proud of the new organization, and proud of Mary Breckinridge. Once again she had received a vote of confidence from the mountain people.

From Katharine E. Wilkie and Elizabeth R. Moseley, Frontier Nurse: Mary Breckinridge *(New York: Simon and Schuster, 1969), 89–97*

PRAISE FOR MARY BRECKINRIDGE

Mary Breckinridge, a Southern belle, born to comfort and pleasure, chose to dedicate her life to a fight against the tragic infant mortality that blighted the lives of the mountain people of Kentucky. Her dream was to create a nursing service that would reach families that never had known the benefits of medicine. With her staff she rode horseback to the most remote cabins and worked under the most primitive conditions. She died at the age of eighty-four, but the Frontier Nursing Service lives on, and with it the memory of an indomitable woman who overcame all odds to turn a humanitarian dream into reality.

From Katharine E. Wilkie and Elizabeth R. Moseley, Frontier Nurse: Mary Breckinridge *(New York: Simon and Schuster, 1969)*

KENTUCKY, 1923

In 1923, Americans drive cars, talk on the telephone, and use electric toasters. Planes fly overhead and people dance to jazz on the radio. But in the Appalachian mountains of Kentucky the twentieth century has not started. People live in tiny cabins without running water. They travel by mule on winding tracks and secret mountain pathways. They eke out hardscrabble livings by farming a little and hunting a little and moonshining, which is against the law. There are no radios. In the evening fiddle music sings through the trees.

The Kentucky mountains are rich with devil's paintbrush and redbud. Before sunrise the valleys fill with clouds. After dark the hollows echo with a chorus of night creatures. . . . But beyond the wildflowers and the sound of the fiddle music, there is much suffering.

From Rosemary Wells, Mary on Horseback *(New York: Viking, 1999),* 7

EARLY MIDWIFERY TRAINING

Mary Breckinridge was director of the Frontier Nursing Service for forty years, and she was a member of a very well known Kentucky family that came in through the Cumberland Gap in [the] late 1700s and went on to settle near Lexington. Mrs. Breckinridge's father was a minister in Russia, and the family lived in Russia all through her girlhood years. However, she went to school in Switzerland. Her brother was born in Russia, delivered by a midwife under the supervision of a doctor.

The Breckinridge family moved back to the United States. Mary married [soon thereafter], but her husband died within a year after their marriage. She decided that she'd like to be a nurse, so she went to St. Luke's in New York and took her general training there, then graduated about 1910. She had two children, Brecky and Polly. Brecky lived to be four and one-half years old, but Polly died about six hours after delivery because she was premature. . . . When Brecky died, that was an awful shock to Mary, so she said that for every hour of Brecky's life she would give the same to a child. She said the rest of her life would be given, not dedicated, to the service of children. Mary's marriage was dissolved and she took her own maiden name back again, thus became Mary Breckinridge.

She went to France with many other wealthy American women to rehabilitate the children, especially those who had lost their parents and starving children in that country. . . . She always used to tell a story that they needed milk very badly, so she wrote to all her friends and told them that she either wanted money to pay for a goat, or she wanted a goat. Well, she went around everywhere, supervising everything, and when she got back to headquarters one day she found twenty-nine goats waiting for her. So the children had enough milk from then on.

After all of that was over she came back to the States and her mother died fairly soon afterwards. When that happened, Mary decided she wanted to do something for the people in her own state. But she knew that in this southeast corner of Kentucky was a part of the country that was more or less isolated and cut off by the mountain barrier. She didn't know very much about it, but she talked to people in Lexington and they suggested she might come up in here and do surveys, seeing really if there was anything that could be done for these people who were secluded.

During the summer, 1923, she spent time up in these mountains going around to the various county seats talking to the judges, any doctors that were there, and all the people, especially important ones. . . . She rode a horse up between Hyden and Beech Fork and came across this beautiful bend in the river and thought it was about four miles from Hyden, so she thought to herself, "If I ever come to Leslie County to live, that's where I'm going to build my house."

That's why Wendover is on that little knoll above the river. She talked to the people, including judges, doctors, and many others, including some local midwives. Due to the remoteness of Leslie County, she thought this would be the best place for her to locate. During that summer she got a friend of hers, Dr. Ella Woodyard, from a Teacher's College in Columbia, to come and survey the Leslie County children, and she did. Dr. Woodyard found that the children of this area were bright, their IQs were just as high as the IQs of anybody outside the area. . . .

One of the first nurses to help Mrs. Breckinridge was a local girl who had gone to someplace in Pennsylvania to get her nurse training. She came back to take care of her father, who had typhoid fever. He died, but his daughter stayed and helped Mrs. Breckinridge.

After the survey was taken in 1923, it helped her to see that local people were self-supporting, with their own farms, cattle, hogs, chickens, gardens, and everything they really wanted except coffee and a few other things like that. The locals were very proud, thus wouldn't accept charity at all. They were self-sufficient, except they had no medical care, so she saw that's where she could help. The maternal mortality rate was very high due to typhoid and diphtheria epidemics and everything else, but there were no doctors to help them out. So she saw that if she could come up in here, that is where she would help.

The local midwives did what they could but didn't do any prenatal work. They just went to the mother when she had her baby. . . . Sometimes nature goes haywire and there is no help for mothers. If you sent for a doctor you'd have to wait about six hours for one to come from Hazard. Consequently the maternal mortality rate was high, so that's where Mrs. Breckinridge thought she could help the children, even before they were born. So she went back to Lexington, where she taught, and then decided that if she were to come up here to work she would have to be a midwife. Well, you couldn't get your midwifery training in the United States in those days, so all babies were delivered by doctors or local women. So she decided she'd better go to Europe to get her midwifery training, which she did.

She went to England and got her midwifery training at the British Hospital for Mothers and Babies. She then went to the General Lying-In Hospital in London and then went to the Central Midwives Board and told them what she wanted to do, because she had to start absolutely from scratch. They were all very good to her and told her all information she needed. From London she went up to Scotland and there met Sir Leslie Mackenzie in Edinburgh, who was head of the Scots nurses, and he suggested she should go up to the Highlands and the islands of the Hebrides to see what the nurses were doing up there. There in the Highlands the mountains are a little bit like they are here in Leslie County, and there in the Highlands the nurses also rode horses or walked through the mountains to get to their patients. She thought that if they could do it up there in Scotland they could do it here.

So she went back to London to get all the information she needed and then came back to the United States. When she got there all the doctors in Lexington were very interested, and all of the specialists gave her a sort of routine that the nurses here would follow. See, we nurses don't prescribe and we don't diagnose. We can make a tentative diagnosis, and we can give that to the doctor, and if there's anything wrong he will tell us how to treat it. Well, in those days we didn't have the wonder drugs that we have now, and we don't [didn't] have all the paraphernalia that they have now to do everything to everybody. It was just a simple way of life.

When Mary was in France she met two nurses where she was working, and these two nurses were going to England to take their midwifery schooling. Since she was so very interested in these nurses, Mary said, "When you are in London and I'm there, too, I would like to meet you and talk to you about your thoughts relative to helping me in Kentucky."

So when they were all in London they got together and these two nurses, Freida Caffin and Edna Rockstroh, decided they would come to Leslie County, Kentucky, with her. So in 1925 Mary Breckinridge and these two nurses came here to live. And the mother of Nurse Caffin came with them.

When they arrived in Hyden, everybody wondered what these women were doing here. Mrs. Breckinridge told all of them, "We're nurses and we're midwives. If you want to come and visit us, please do, and also bring your children. So if we can help you in any way, we will. If you bring your children and they've got sores or anything, we'll help. . . . And, of course, you can come and visit us and we'd like to visit with you, but we are not coming into your homes unless you invite us." People began to think these women knew what they were talking about, and they would talk to the nurses and everybody got to know everybody.

It takes a while to get people's confidence, because they don't know what you're doing. They wondered how the new nurses knew how to take care of a woman when she was having a baby. But very soon they got to realize that these nurses did know what they were talking about. Of course, Mrs. Breckinridge ran things with her own money for the first few months, but she couldn't do that for very long, so she had to go outside to get money to get the Frontier Nursing Service going. And rather than stay in Hyden all her service time, she wanted to cover at least one thousand square miles. So she went out to form committees in the various eastern states. So we went to Louisville, Lexington, Boston, New York, Chicago, Detroit, Washington, all those places. They formed committees, and people got very interested in the service, and she never once asked for money. She always told them what the conditions were and what we were doing, and money just came in for support. Before she started to build a center, people came to her and said, "We want you to come to us," and she would say, "Well, we have to do something about it. You get the people together and talk about it and then I'll come; and tell them if they decide they want us to come where you are, we'll see what we can do about it."

She then built service outposts at Beech Fork, Confluence, Red Bird, Flat Creek, Burlington, and Burgess. She also got the money from various persons for a hospital to be built on the hill, a hospital that had twelve beds and some bassinets. In June 1928, Sir Leslie and Lady Mackenzie came over from Scotland to dedicate it. After that we were soon able to get a part-time doctor who served public health and the Frontier Nursing Service, both part-time. We were also having some midwifery services by that time. Then, in 1931, the Depression hit us, and when it did people couldn't send us any money after that, because they had [to] do all they could to keep their own house. So the FNS got to be very poor, but we didn't close down, we just managed. Some of the nurses had to leave and some of us stayed. We didn't have any money, but we were very happy. We had enough to eat and a bed to sleep on and our horses were taken care of. When we got out of the Depression we went on and founded the Graduate School of Midwifery in 1939.

Excerpted from an account told by Betty Lester, Hyden, to Jonathan Freid, March 3, 1978; provided by the Louie B. Nunn Center for Oral History, University of Kentucky Libraries, Lexington

MARY BRECKINRIDGE AS MOTIVATOR

Mrs. Breckinridge motivated people to have faith in what was going on. First of all there was herself. She truly inspired faith herself as she went around because she recognized that she had to sell herself and her services to the people. She liked them and they liked her, and that was the start of it all. In creating a new district for Frontier Nursing Service she would send Mary Willeford and Gladys Peacock, who were in charge of the building operations and setting up nursing districts while getting to know people. That was their main purpose. Of course, they also did top-notch nursing and also were excellent midwives.

When they got a new district going, Mrs. Breckinridge had some nurses that she was ready to put into it, and they moved on when Willeford and Peacock opened another district. Their work wasn't on any regular schedule. They didn't say, "This week we'll open this one, and next month we'll open that one." Of course, there wasn't a certain amount of demand. Of course, Mrs. Breckinridge helped to create that demand, too, because she would have committee meetings and it wouldn't be too long before the people were wanting to have a nursing district in their community.

There was no effort on the part of the community to finance what was going on because the fees were so nominal that they really made very little contribution. However, at the same time there was a gesture that implied Mrs. Breckinridge had faith that these people did want to pay their way. The locals also helped with building efforts, especially during earlier years, while I was there.

During my first term there they celebrated their tenth anniversary, and I think that all centers had been built by that time except some that have been established very recently. While I was there the Frontier Nursing Service was the only health care system in operation.

Told by Dorothy Caldwell, Burlington, to Marion Barrett, January 18, 1979; provided by the Louie B. Nunn Center for Oral History, University of Kentucky Libraries, Lexington

MARY BRECKINRIDGE FELL OFF A HORSE

I'll tell you about what happened to Mary Breckinridge, who fell in November 1932 and broke her back while riding a horse called Traveler. Mary had been out on tour, and while she was away Leona Morgan asked me if we would buy a bluegrass horse, that she was very much interested in us buying that horse and bringing it up to try him out. I said, "Leona, we don't have the money for a new horse and we don't need one."

"Well, just try him, he's beautiful," she said.

Well, it was hard to turn locals down when they were trying to be helpful, so I said, "All right, we'll take him on a two-weeks trial under the agreement, but don't get your heart set on our buying him."

So everybody wanted to ride that horse in the next two weeks, and even I rode and tried him out. That horse had a beautiful gait and was young, with a nice personality. We all wanted to buy him, but we didn't have the $150 in the budget that was asked for him. So one of us conceived the idea that maybe the staff could buy the horse for Mrs. Breckinridge to replace her horse, Teddy Bear. If you read her book, *Wide Neighborhoods*, you will know that she was very fond of Teddy Bear, that had fallen off a cliff and had to be destroyed.

She never replaced Teddy Bear, and so we decided that at the Thanksgiving dinner at the hospital that year we would give the new horse to Mrs. Breckinridge. She had come in and she thought the new horse was great and mentioned that he was more like Teddy Bear than the horse that had replaced Teddy Bear. So we all got together at the Thanksgiving dinner and she told us she had already named the new horse Traveler and that it was a good name for him. She told us that she was going out soon after that on her fall tour. We all went to the barn for her mount onto the horse.

It was on a Sunday afternoon, and the courier was there and the girl who was taking the pack mule back. So everything was ready, but it was beginning to drizzle and Mrs. Breckinridge had on her riding raincoat, which was a cape type of thing, that is, a coat with a cape-type thing over it so you could put your arms through the slit in the coat. Mrs. Breckinridge never buttoned the coat, she just let it flop. She got on Traveler and started off. As she rode off I turned to her secretary, Wilma, and said, "Wilma, isn't it a comfort to see her get on a safe horse?"

Well, the next thing we knew, halfway up Hurricane Mrs. Breckinridge threw herself off because she realized that Traveler was running away, but she wasn't, and she didn't have the proper bittings to control him, so she picked the least rocky place along the road under those circumstances. When she threw herself off, two of her back vertebras were crushed.

The car waiting for her at the head of Hurricane was to take her to Hazard but took her back to Hyden. She didn't lose consciousness but threw herself in front of a house, and when some mountain men came out to help her she told them exactly how to lift her and what to do, so they put her in the back of the car and took her up to the hospital. Then, the next day, the undertakers in Lexington sent an ambulance for her from Hazard, but an ambulance from Hazard couldn't get up the big hill, so they sent a hearse, as I remember. They took her down to the Lafayette Hotel, where the doctors put her on a Bradford frame in the hotel and there she stayed. . . .

When all that was completed, Mrs. Breckinridge couldn't come home until she could ride a horse. So we sent Carminettie, just a pony really, and Kermit Morgan to lead her. Mrs. Breckinridge had a rubber cushion to sit on, and Kermit was to just lead the pony as slowly as possible down the creek to her house.

That was a terrible experience! [Laughter.]

Told by Agnes Lewis, Maryville, TN, to Dale Deaton,
January 5, 1979; provided by the Louie B. Nunn Center
for Oral History, University of Kentucky Libraries, Lexington

HARD TIMES DURING DEPRESSION YEARS

When the Depression got so bad that we could not meet the salaries, Mrs. Breckinridge called the staff members together and said that she would let any members of the staff leave who had to leave, but those who were willing to [could] stay on and take what pay they could get until she got things. Well, she was always optimistic, and she expected to get things straightened out soon. And anyone who had family responsibilities and could not live on uncertainty would be paid. I think three members left and the others stayed on. . . . Theoretically, Mrs. Breckinridge cut all the salaries by one-third, but we were to keep up with the third salary owing everyone, because she was so sure that that was to be paid back. She never would admit that she couldn't meet that obligation. . . .

I think it was during the 1950s when Mrs. Breckinridge went out, and at that point we'd gotten the salaries back up to where the key people—nurses, secretaries, and Mrs. Breckinridge—were getting all of $125 a month. And out of that we paid $40 room and board. When Mrs. Breckinridge went away, Brownie, Betty, Lucille Rogers, and I put our heads together and decided while she was away we would do away with the one-third salary that was due everybody and that we would straighten things out and pay everybody $125 whenever we could raise it. Well, when Mrs. Breckinridge came back we told her with fear and trembling what we had decided, and I think she was relieved. Of course, she said she never could have gone back on her word. We knew that, and that's the reason we did it.

All during World War II, I spent most of my time writing firms and saying, "I enclose our check for so much, as this is all we can pay, but we'll pay you more when we can." And just by sending a little bit each month, which was a nuisance, and keeping up with the rest of it, we kept the accounts open, but we never failed to write them that letter. Of course, we did pay the wages, but they were low during the war. The executive committee wanted to close some of the [medical] centers, but Mrs. Breckinridge would not do it. She always wondered what would happen to the buildings if that were done, so she didn't allow it. . . . Of course, she went ahead and sent the money, and we had the house recovered. That was in the late 1940s.

She truly wanted things to go on the right way. She did know how to give up, but in her mind she wouldn't do it. I don't remember her questioning the purchase of any equipment or supplies that were absolutely necessary for the hospital. However, she expected our doctor and our nurses to know how to get along with the minimum. She didn't want any fancy gadgets around, but they did use some things like incubators, which you brought immature babies through, along with hot water bottles and lamps, and they were great!

> *Told by Agnes Lewis, Maryville, TN, to Dale Deaton,*
> *January 5, 1979; provided by the Louie B. Nunn Center*
> *for Oral History, University of Kentucky Libraries, Lexington*

1940s Flu Epidemic

Back in the 1940s we had a flu epidemic here in Wendover, and all staff members at Wendover were in the hospital being treated in bed, with very high temperatures. All hospital staff members were over at Wendover halfway house until they could go back on duty. Just routinely, we had Walter Begley lined up to bring his truck in, go to the hospital and pick up those who were ready to convalesce, then bring them to Wendover, where we had all Wendover patients who had gotten sick in the middle of the night and had high temperatures. Thus they were ready to go over to the hospital and be put to bed. Of course, we spent most of our time changing beds and taking care of the sick.

Mrs. Breckinridge, Dorothy Buck, and I were the only ones at Wendover who didn't take the flu. Mrs. Breckinridge called me and Bucket [Buck] in and said to us, "Have you packed your overnight bag for the hospital?"

We said, "No, we haven't." Then she said, "Then go and do it. I packed the last one that I'm gonna pack." And so Bucket and I left and we went and put nighties, dressing gowns, and toothbrushes in and were ready. But we never used it. Then, believe me, a few months after that I came down with flu and was in bed for two weeks. I said, "Well, I just didn't want to have it when I couldn't get any attention." But this time I got plenty attention.

That was a critical situation, about having to close parts of the Frontier Nursing Service for a time during that epidemic. Of course, everybody at the hospital went around with masks on, and they used the best technique they knew to prevent spreading anything. The nurses did, too, but they had to go out when they had no business going on in the hospital.

> *Told by Agnes Lewis, Maryville, TN, to Dale Deaton,*
> *January 5, 1979; provided by the Louie B. Nunn Center for*
> *Oral History, University of Kentucky Libraries, Lexington*

Origin of FNS Graduate School of Midwifery

The Frontier Nursing School of Midwifery was founded under the leadership of Mary Breckinridge, and World War II really necessitated it. . . . The plan that Mrs. Breckinridge originally had [back around 1939] was to have a school that would be affiliated with University of Kentucky, . . . and students would take some of their training in Lexington and some of the fieldwork here. That's the only way I've heard about its origin. During World War II, I went to Lexington with Mrs. Breckinridge when she was on her way to speak in New York. While sitting in the railroad station waiting for a train, she suddenly turned to me and said, "Oh, by the way, I don't think I told you that on my trip I'm going to tell [various] committees that we have to start our midwifery school right now in the hospital."

Well, the hospital was bursting at the seams then, as every available room had been converted into a clinic or office or something. I could just see the confusion caused by incorporating a school, but that's what she said. Sometime during that year Nora Kelly was pulled in from the district at Confluence and was put in charge of two students who were the first ones in the midwifery graduate school.

I'll tell you that the tension of times over there was pretty awful, with the school running and everybody crowded and piled on top [of each other]. But it was done, and I think they had it ready in about two years. When it opened we trained two Indian girls, and that was very good for us but it was difficult. One of them was a Cherokee and was a very attractive young Indian lady. She later married an agricultural demonstration agent at Hazard and lives there to this day. She was most attractive in her riding habit and could ride like the wind. . . . The other Indian girl was Virginia, but I've forgotten what tribe she was with, but she was very silent. She had to be placed in an outpost center with another nurse, which was hard on that other nurse because this Indian girl would not communicate. She simply went out on district service, took good care of her patients, and that was fine. However, once they got home she went to her room and even during meals she would sit in utter silence.

> *Told by Agnes Lewis, Maryville, TN, to Dale Deaton,*
> *January 5, 1979; provided by the Louie B. Nunn Center for*
> *Oral History, University of Kentucky Libraries, Lexington*

Trouble Driving a Jeep

On the application I was asked, "Can you drive?" Actually, I was thinking more about horseback riding, but driving jeeps was probably as important, but since Agnes Lewis did not drive, I drove on a number of occasions to take her around to various outpost centers and into Hazard to do various chores she had to do. She was a little bit frightened on the road because of the steep embankments, and I could tell she was a little nervous.

I was a new driver and had learned to drive within the last year before I came to Wendover. Well, due to all the precipitous curves and going off the road onto bumpy mountainous roads and then having to turn around and back up was a scary situation. I would invariably get into trouble going through back-up situations and then turning to go forward. If you back into a low place and then you were going to pull out you had to change into four-wheel drive, and whenever I went through the gears to get into four-wheel drive I would forget to get out of reverse, and then I would go sailing farther down the hill than I had before.

On one notable occasion when another courier and I went out [to] the movies one evening and the jeep was parked out in the tin garage at the highway, she opened the garage doors for me and I backed the jeep out onto the highway. I happened to go slightly off the shoulder on the side of the road, so I thought I'd better get into four-wheel drive in order to pull up on the road. Of course, as usual, I forgot to get out of reverse, and the next thing I knew I had gone way off down this very steep embankment and almost ran into the river.

Of course, when she put down the garage door and turned around to look up the road and down the road but couldn't see me, since I had disappeared. She had no idea where I was, and I was clinging on for dear life way down the embankment, probably twenty-five or thirty yards down this very steep embankment, which was almost a vertical drop into the river. We were almost two feet from the river in what was likely the major Wendover jeep. Here comes another jeep down the road and, as typical, the driver had a chain in the jeep for pulling purposes. So with both jeeps in a four-wheel drive we were soon up on the highway and on our way to the movie in Hyden.

> *Told by Carolyn Booth Gregory, Evanston, IL, to Linda Green,*
> *March 31, 1979; provided by the Louie B. Nunn Center for*
> *Oral History, University of Kentucky Libraries, Lexington*

VISITING WITH THE LOCAL PEOPLE

On numerous occasions when Agnes Lewis and I were out on errands, I had numerous opportunities to meet some of the mountain families and just to sit and talk and get to know the concerns of the local people and learn how much they really did revere the Frontier Nursing Services. Of course, we often talked about very small problems and things, such as how the agricultural crops were going, how quilt making was going, whether or not the Middle Fork River had risen too much for the kids to get in school, and just minor health problems that somebody had, such as colds, fevers, and those sorts of things.

The nurses were always concerned about the elderly people and whether or not their homes were insulated and warm and what more could be done to make their homes more comfortable. And I know the nurses were always admonishing them about the fireplaces and the little girls that were running around in scanty clothes. Little girls seemed to get burned in the fireplace much more than the boys, and I know Mrs. Breckinridge, before she died, was very happy to see the new era come in when little girls wore jeans as well as little boys.

Visits in the homes were one of the most enjoyable parts of my stay, and in getting to know the people better.

> *Told by Carolyn Booth Gregory, Evanston, IL, to Linda Green,*

March 31, 1979; provided by the Louie B. Nunn Center for
Oral History, University of Kentucky Libraries, Lexington

INTRODUCTION TO FNS

Back in 1935 I came to the Frontier Nursing Service because my father was a surgeon and had gone there to teach some volunteer clinic work. He came back home from there and said that he had been in a place that he knew I would like to go and put in some work time. Everything sounded good, based on what he said about it. I didn't know anything about it, but his description of it turned me on. He told about the nurses there and said that none of them were American nurses and that they were all British.

I asked if I could become a courier there, and they sent me a form to fill out and then I was interviewed by an ex-courier here in Cincinnati. The fact that I went there as a courier and became a part of life that was different from anything else that I had ever known was just great. [Leslie County] was where the main economic activity at that time was farming, and I loved to ride horses.

Told by Dorothy Caldwell, Burlington, to Marion Barrett,
January 18, 1979; provided by the Louie B. Nunn Center for
Oral History, University of Kentucky Libraries, Lexington

DYING MAN DIDN'T DIE

Some of the things that really endeared me to the Frontier Nursing Service were the outrageous things they would ask people to do. A vivid example is about the time I was working at the Cincinnati General Hospital in the nursing office and Agnes Lewis telephoned me at home one night and said that she was going to make a request of me, that she hoped I would be able to help them out. She told me about a patient from Frontier Nursing Service who had been sent to Cincinnati for treatment and care, and that he would not live long. She also asked me if I would find out which one of them would be cheaper; that is, to let him die and send his body back or send an ambulance to bring him home to die.

I couldn't think of any way to find that out, so I just chuckled, since I thought that was the most unbelievable thing. Anyway, every morning when I first came to work my first duty came to be to go to the information desk and ask how the patient was doing. Well, he lived!

The problem became less pressing, and it was no longer "let's get this found out quickly before he dies and there is no alternative left but to take him in as a body." That bothered me, because I couldn't figure out a way to find out about that poor man that was dying. I almost thought I was failing him, but luckily he lived, and so he solved it for me!

Told by Dorothy Caldwell, Burlington, to Marion Barrett,
January 19, 1979; provided by the Louie B. Nunn Center for
Oral History, University of Kentucky Libraries, Lexington

PIONEER NURSING ACTIVITIES

Mary Breckinridge was involved with the nurse-midwife activities from the word go. First of all, she started this now here, the first organized group of midwives. But then she was on the committee for the standard-ization of midwifery in New York City with Dr. Loganstein. Mary was a great friend of Hazel Corbin, who headed Maternity Center in those days but was not a midwife. Hazel Corbin was interested in improving the welfare of mothers and children. When Maternity Center decided they should start a midwifery school, she allowed Rose McNaught to go from here to New York to help them get it under way, and they have always been grateful. Now the present-day director of Maternity Center Association, Ruth [?], has just written a thesis on midwifery for her doctorate, and anything that she writes and she always gives credit to Mary Breckinridge for setting the pattern of midwifery in this county, but she's a fighter too.

I think the important thing is that it's always been organizations that have been the pioneers in the health field. Now they're becoming more and more standardized underneath the government, so who's going to pioneer now?

Told by Helen E. Browne, Wendover, to Dale Deaton,
March 27, 1979; provided by the Louie B. Nunn Center for
Oral History, University of Kentucky Libraries, Lexington

RED CROSS VOLUNTEERS IN WORLD WAR II

The volunteers and the couriers who took the Red Cross Emergency Nurses Training and the work they did during World War II was tremendous. We wouldn't have been able to keep the hospital open without them. Because I was in the hospital then, at the peak in time during which we were shortest of nurses. Frequently I was the only registered nurse on the floor during the day taking care of the mothers and babies. But I had to sort of look out for the other side of general patients. So many times the nurses were a great help. Number one, these were volunteers that had already been down and done their service as couriers, and they realized that we were awfully short of nursing help, so they went up to the Red Cross facility. However, the advantage was that they already knew these people and had become very fond of them. Otherwise they never would have done this, to come back and help. So the local people related to them extremely well when they were in the hospital, and I think they were well-trained, intelligent girls, and they used their own imaginations. I would go over and look at the patients in the morning, and we always had a nurse on night duty, which was a saving grace.

And we also had spells where we didn't have any registered nurses except me during the day, so I used to go over to see the general patients every morning and take care of them with the aides. Then we had to put out a plea for nurses to come and maybe give us a month or two.

We had one elderly woman as a patient who was really sick. And we had a young aide on with her, and we also had a child very sick with typhoid fever. The little girl's temperature would spike up to 106 degrees but plummet down to 95 degrees, and the aide didn't want this child to get a low temperature, so she decided to pack her in ice bags. The aide came on one morning and came rushing to me and said, "I can't get her temperature to register at all."

I went over and the poor little thing was freezing, so I told the aide to take the ice packs away. Then I looked at the nurse and said, "You know, the temperature is so low the girl can't cope, so that's an awfully dangerous thing to do."

She said, "I don't want it to come up again."

I said, "Well, just keep her cold all the time." But it was the aide who realized this was a dangerous thing, you see, so she came running. [No conclusion to the story.]

*Told by Helen E. Browne, Wendover, to Dale Deaton,
March 27, 1979; provided by the Louie B. Nunn Center for
Oral History, University of Kentucky Libraries, Lexington*

NURSE'S DEVOTED HORSE

This took place back in 1939 or '40. Back then the fireplace was the only warm place in the house on a cold day. When you went on a delivery during cold weather you would burn in the front and freeze in the back, and then you had to stand around and burn up your back and freeze in front. I've drawn beds across the room near to the fireplace to keep the mother warm. We had bad winters back then, because I was on Bull Creek Clinic, when you had to ride over Thousandsticks Mountain, located behind the hospital.

It was horseback days back then, and I walked nearly a mile, since I could take my horse quite happily as far as the old Bull Creek Clinic, which was at the mouth of Thousandsticks, but I had to walk from there. One night I had gone on a delivery, and I had ridden a horse up from Osmond's Fork to Getty Bowling's house. When I got there I said to him, "Now, you've got to come out and walk my horse every half hour or so, just walk him around. I'll leave the saddle on the horse but I'll loosen the girth, because he's going to get cold."

The Bowlings had their own mule in the barn, and I wouldn't have turned that down for my horse for anything. So Mr. Bowling did quite faithfully until he got excited, until the baby was born, so I looked up and said, "What about my horse?"

He went out and came back and said, "Miss Browne, the horse is gone." My horse had slipped his bridle and off he'd gone.

So when I finished what I was doing he had a mule that was a slowpoke, and I said, "Well, Getty, I can't carry these big heavy delivery bags, so I want you to come with me as far as Bull Creek Clinic and I'll lock them up in the closet and then walk home from there."

It was a bright, moonlight night, so he did, but he was a little bit worried about me going, so I said, "No, no, it's a bright, moonlight night, and I'm not afraid of anything." So I took off and told him he could go home. When I got to the foot of the hill down to the hospital I heard my horse, so I whistled to him. Well, he waited. He was very embarrassed. Fortunately, I had taken the bridle with me, but he was waiting for me with his head down. So he let me put the bridle on, and I was glad to have a horse to ride up and over the hill.

Told by Helen E. Browne, Wendover, to Dale Deaton,
March 27, 1979; provided by the Louie B. Nunn Center for
Oral History, University of Kentucky Libraries, Lexington

EARLY NURSING AT HYDEN

I've often been asked, "How did you ever come to Leslie County?" It was so remote at that time that there was not a foot of railroad nor automobile road, and of course no electricity at that time in 1918. I met Miss Lila Byers, the sister of Reverend Byers of the Presbyterian Church in Hyden. She and I became friends, and she told me about the work she was doing as a schoolteacher, matron, in the girls' dormitory, and also a Bible teacher in the church.

There was no nurse in the county at that time, and no hospital. The only two doctors were very often not available. . . . While this was going on, Lila Byers's sister-in-law had contacted the Public Health Department in Louisville and asked if they would send the director of public health nurses in Kentucky to Leslie County and appeal to the fiscal court to help support a public health nurse for Leslie County. And the director did speak to the fiscal court, and they agreed to pay twenty-five dollars a month to Nurse Smiley. The Red Cross was also to pay twenty-five dollars, and the state of Kentucky was to pay the other twenty-five dollars. And then Miss Williamson, the director of nurses in Louisville, said, "I don't know where I could ever find a nurse to travel these sixteen miles from the railroad at Crypton and into this remote area."

It was then that Miss Lila Byers told her sister-in-law of having met me in Chicago, and they wrote to the Public Health Department. The Health Department then wrote me and asked if I would consider coming and if I would come by Louisville to the office of the Public Health Department for an interview. Well, I did that, and that's the story as to why I went to work in Leslie County.

Told by Jean Tolk, Barbourville, to Dale Deaton,
November 1, 1978; provided by the Louie B. Nunn Center for
Oral History, University of Kentucky Libraries, Lexington

WARREN COUNTY'S FIRST REGISTERED NURSE

This is an oral history interview with Shella and Alice Procter, who were nieces of Ms. Ora Porter, a black lady who was Warren County's first registered nurse.

Ora Porter was a social person who enjoyed her clubs, meetings, and church activities. . . . The furnishings in her home were Victorian in nature, and she liked to keep things just as they were. She often shared her afternoons with Shella and Alice by taking them on walks through the town of Bowling Green.

Shella knew her when Ora nursed their sick uncle in Russellville for four weeks. The sisters and parents lived at that time in Auburn, and often their father would rent a car and go visit Ora and other friends in Bowling Green. Shella's family and especially her mother were as close to Ora as anyone. Shella's mother sewed for Ora, sometimes making her uniforms and dresses, and took care of Ora when she had surgery in Nashville.

Most of the relatives outside of Shella's immediate family lived in different parts of Kentucky, or in Indianapolis or New York City. Julius was the only surviving nephew, of three until recently. The two other brothers had died long ago. One of them died in a tobacco factory that was blown down by the wind in Bowling Green.

Shella and Alice lived in Bowling Green during the years 1927–1929, during which time they attended an all-black high school called State Street High School. The first year they lived with a Mrs. Jackson and became accustomed to the size and newness of Bowling Green. Thus they were not very excited when they came to live with Ora during the second two years of attending high school. . . . Living with Aunt Ora could be difficult at times, depending upon her moods. Ora was obsessed with neatness and cleanliness, and it was the nieces' job to keep the house just "so, so . . ."

Ora did travel often in the United States during the winter months. She would sometimes visit Tuskegee, at which she had earlier received her nurse's degree. A male friend there gave her a gold band, which she much later entrusted to Shella. Whether it was the friend who had asked her to marry him is unknown, but Ora had always remained single. . . .

Ora worked long hours as a "call nurse" in the homes of white patrons in the area. She often stayed on cases for extended periods of time, such as ten to twelve weeks or as long as the patient needed her. She was very seldom home, and when she was she would get busy with duties around the house and yard.

She was not a hospital-assigned nurse but would often accompany a private patient into the hospital. She never talked about her patients, just as doctors didn't do it either. However, we do know that most of her patients were white. This was similar to the sister's father's situation. Being a tailor, his clients were mainly white, because they were the people who could afford it. Very few blacks could afford it in those days.

Typhoid was a common occurrence in the area, especially during the summer months. Alice equated its frequency to that of tuberculosis, which was also common. Ora Porter was known as an excellent typhoid nurse, partly because of her ability to come in and put the affected household in order. She would take over and lay the rules down whenever she went to someone's home. She would see to it that the home was completely sanitized and a relaxed, quiet environment was established for the patient. She was particular about the patient's diet and would often prepare the food herself.

Shella and Alice do not remember a specific typhoid epidemic, such as that reported in the early 1920s in Auburn, Kentucky. The sisters instead think of typhoid as being a very common event.

Ora possibly worked with Dr. Blackburn, although little is remembered about him. Likewise, not much is known of her association with Dr. Porter (a distant cousin of Ora) and Dr. Jones. Alice noted, however, that Ora nursed her when Dr. Porter was testing her for menorrhagia [menstrual disorder] when she lived with Ora. Alice said she had a problem swallowing pills and that Ora "gave me the devil after that, but now I take them by the half-dozen and don't think anything about it."

Ora had the reputation of being the best. Because of this she was busy most of the time working as a private nurse. She was paid by the day, somewhere between fifteen and twenty dollars each day.

In trying to determine how long Ora was a nurse, the sisters concluded that she had been a nurse even before they were born.

Told by Robert J. Gates, Cincinnati, OH, to Shella Procter and Alice Procter, Russellville, February 26, 1992; provided by the Special Collections Library, Western Kentucky University, Bowling Green.

Young Girl Never Met Mary Breckinridge

My earliest memories of the Frontier Nursing Service were to hear my mother talking about it. My mother had gotten involved with the FNS through Mrs. Breckinridge. She knew Mrs. Breckinridge through her brother, General James Breckinridge, and they met before the war was over down in Paris Island.

Mrs. Breckinridge was a friend of my grandmother, and that's how my mother met all of them. And at that time my mother was writing books, and she asked Mrs. Breckinridge if she could sometime go down to Wendover, because she wanted to write a book about it, and she did.

I think she met Mrs. Breckinridge in 1947, and I think she spent about a month down there, or six weeks.

I don't know when I started remembering, but always my mother talked about Mary Breckinridge, but I always remember having a horse at age three, and it was always my big dream to go down there and meet Mrs. Breckinridge. You know, riding horses back then was a part of the FNS. Things didn't work out, though, so I never did meet Mary Breckinridge. She died before I ever went to Wendover.

Told by Mary Lansing to Anne Campbell Ritchie,
November 30, 1970; provided by the Louie B. Nunn Center
for Oral History, University of Kentucky Libraries, Lexington

SCARED BY NURSE'S ACTIVITY

I remember once when I was at an outpost center with a young child who had had an appendectomy. And they had like a draining spoon, but I don't recall what the technical term is. I was standing there with the nurse on one side of the table, and the little child and I were on the other side.

[The nurse] started fooling around with the spoon, and I passed out! I had never passed out in my life, but I realized then and there I would never make it in terms of being a nurse or a doctor.

Told by Mary Lansing to Anne Campbell Ritchie,
November 30, 1970; provided by the Louie B. Nunn Center
for Oral History, University of Kentucky Libraries, Lexington

FRIENDLY, HELPFUL MIDWIVES

My grandmother was fantastic! She delivered me, so I came out okay! She was a midwife and highly approved of the nurse-midwives. Eventually they took care of her. That was the best service I have ever seen, even when my grandmother was in bed. She stayed at my son's about one year because she got to the place where she wasn't thinking really good, but she still knew what was going on. She was eighty-four when she passed away.

Miss Joy Bloomfield and another nurse would come every day, so I complimented them one day. We always tried to have coffee or cake or something. That was a nice time for us, since we were teenagers then. Well, actually, I was married then, and I just thanked the nurses one day for what they had done for my mom, and for my grandmother.

They said, "It's not us, it's your mother, Ollie, that's doing all this." Of course, she had gotten to the place where she was just in bed, more like a child. But they always came, because they were friends.

Told by Georgia Ledford to Carol Crowe-Carraco,
August 17, 1978; provided by the Louie B. Nunn Center
for Oral History, University of Kentucky Libraries, Lexington

SERVICES PERFORMED ON HORSEBACK

When I came to Hyden in 1937 as a courier, we took a bus from Lexington to Hazard. From there we took another bus to Hyden. When you're halfway to Hyden you get off at the head of Hurricane Creek, where someone meets you with a horse. Then you ride a horse four miles down to the service, carrying a little suitcase on a horse.

When I got to where I was going, I was met by Jean Holmes, who was head courier [and] who stayed in the old garden house. All the couriers stayed there. Well, Mary Breckinridge was also there, since she had broken her back and wasn't traveling very much right then. She'd go out to meetings and things, but in the meantime she'd stay in her bedroom, where she'd have meetings. People would go up to see her, and I saw her every day at lunch.

We always took care of the horses, since we had six or eight in the barn. The nurses had their own horse, and if we went to an outpost we'd go by horse. So we took just what we could, such as medicines, in our saddlebags to the clinic.

Told by Fredericka Holdship to Dale Deaton, March 25, 1979;
provided by the Louie B. Nunn Center for Oral History,
University of Kentucky Libraries, Lexington

RELAXATION TIMES FOR NURSES

While I was at Wendover there was very little playing around by nurses. It was too difficult. I mean, they were on call both day and night. And if they wanted a weekend, then they'd have to put in something like a weekend and get someone to come to help. If there were two of them, the other one could take over.

Most of the centers did have two nurses at that time. If not, they'd just get one of the floating nurses to come and take over, then they'd take a weekend and go to Lexington, or elsewhere, to visit friends.

It was too hard to get around in those days. Sometimes they just rode over here to spend a few days at Wendover.

Told by Fredericka Holdship to Dale Deaton, March 25, 1979;
provided by the Louie B. Nunn Center for Oral History,
University of Kentucky Libraries, Lexington

2

EMERGENCY ROOM EPISODES

It is hard to imagine how health care was provided and emergencies were handled, if at all, during the early years of our nation, especially in rural communities, small towns, and remote backcountry areas. Due to the lack of doctors, nurses, and hospitals in those areas, healing was at times successfully provided by locals using folk remedies. Disastrous injuries, difficult births, and other emergencies often resulted in physical disability or death. Thus, as local health care became more readily available, with better access to doctors, nurses, and midwives, life became more satisfactory and productive.

Most of the stories in this chapter describe cases in which a patient likely would not have survived without medical services; some didn't. These accounts describe some of the wide range of challenges nurses have to contend with, from handling violent, confused, and inebriated patients, to dealing with uncertainties and mistakes, to managing patients' family members and doctors, to the speed and volume of the work, to witnessing death and the outcome of tragic accidents. Virtually all these stories illustrate the importance of emergency rooms and their staff in Kentucky hospitals.

NURSE RIDES ON PATIENT'S BACK

When I was working in an emergency room in Louisville I was triaging a man who was slightly nuts. He told his name and said he was a Civil War veteran. He had been off his meds for a while and was a little psychotic. The secretary was sitting at her desk and I was taking his blood pressure when all of a sudden he jumped out of the chair and flung himself at the secretary, grabbed her around the neck, and started choking her.

The emergency room doctor was about forty years old and weighed maybe 120 pounds and was about five feet and three inches tall. We were all trying to get this fellow under control without success. Security persons were also there. The emergency room doctor jumped on his back and started saying to this fellow that he was going [down]. Well, this fellow was running around like a bronco trying to shake the doctor off his back. That fellow was about six feet and five inches tall and weighed about 250 pounds. It was the funniest sight you've ever seen with that little woman riding on that huge man's back and telling him he was going down.

We did eventually get him down but it took large doses of Haldol and Thorazine injections through his clothes with that doctor on his back!

Marilyn Kaye Montell, Louisville, August 1, 2010

Dealing with a Naked Man

Another time . . . I was out front in triage when all of a sudden a naked man came running out of the doors from the monitor room where we kept all the heart patients. He had been brought in by ambulance and had escaped from the back of the ambulance, stripped naked, and was trying to get away. He was high on drugs and alcohol.

Where I was located, out front, was where the family and patients waited to visit or be seen by the doctor. There was a huge picture window in the waiting area and it was daylight outside. Well, he came running out through the window that just had an opening. Just as he hit the window he bounced off like a bird and then ran out the door as naked as a jaybird, with the emergency room nurses right behind him trying to catch him.

It was so funny when he got outside to the highway and cars started hitting their breaks and blowing their horns. Finally the police got him, put his clothes back on him, and brought him back in for treatment.

Marilyn Kaye Montell, Louisville, August 1, 2010

The Miracle

One of the scariest parts of being a nurse is the unknown as to what will happen next. Of course, during my many years of being a nurse I never felt totally 100 percent confident that I was going to have a great night on the twelve-hour night shifts. I had a good reason to feel that way during many nights, but one I recall stands out in my mind.

I arrived at work at 7:00 p.m. and started getting a report from the other shift. I was told that my ICU [intensive care unit] patient was really sick but she was doing better. She had been admitted with GI [gastrointestinal] bleeding. Her vital signs were stable. She was alert and oriented, moved all extremities, and had general weakness. A full report was taken, then I walked into the room to the haunting "unknown." I introduced myself to her nurse and initially she responded. Then all of a sudden she started to moan, vomited projectile[s of] bright-red blood, and her eyes rolled back into her lids.

Calling for help, all the night-shift and day-shift crew were in that room as well as doctors who were making rounds. IV bags were being hung while vital signs were taken. New IV access was attempted as doctors gave emergency orders, and staff members [were] running to get blood and [to get] family informed. Permits were signed leading up to intubation. Whew!

What a night, but it was only about 9:00 p.m. What did the rest of the night have in store? It was constant monitoring, new meds to give, comfort measures, and keeping the patient still. Thank goodness I didn't get a new patient admission or have another patient. I kept the IV going, thanks to a central line put in by the doctor, and more blood was given. Blood levels remained in check.

The patient woke up soon after the intubation but was unusually calm when compared to some patients who do not know what is happening. To the best of my ability I explained what had happened and the woman nodded at me as if she understood all that had taken place. With some comfort measures and light sedation the woman did well the rest of the night.

At 7:00 a.m. the oncoming shift took [my] report and I was on my way to my daytime bed. That was one of those bad nights out of many that I recall, but it was worth it. That lady made it to discharge and to her home. However, she did return to say thank you to all the staff that "saved her life."

What a nice ending to the unknown course of a night in nursing. But what I knew deep down, as I did most nights, is that I wasn't the only nurse on duty. I had my team there with me. We were the cohesive night crew along with the helpful day crew, mending hearts together with the hand of God by our side helping us to perform a miracle.

I wasn't at work when that lady patient returned to say her "thank you," but oh, what a blessing to be a part of her care.

Rebecca Collins, Auburn, September 14, 2011

SURGERY WITNESSED

The first night we were at the hospital we were awakened in the middle of the night by someone who announced that a surgeon was preparing to perform an intestinal obstruction on a man who had shown up in the emergency room very sick and very drunk. The not-so-smart surgeon decided it would be a good idea for the new students to see their first surgery. So we were rushed to the OR [operating room], were given masks, ushered to a corner, and told to stay there and not move until the surgery was complete.

The surgeon was very informative as he explained what he was doing while performing the surgery. When the surgery was completed and the wound dressed we were ushered out. I made it to the door and the world went black. The combination of no food the night before, standing in one spot without moving for an hour, the excitement, and the number of bodies so close together was more than my poor body could take.

Ruth A. Buzzard, Dawson Springs, February 23, 2012

AN EARLY ALCOHOLIC EVENT

The day following my first night hospital service I was assigned to a group of patients on the surgical unit. I went to the utility room to obtain some supplies and standing there in the door was a man dressed in a hospital gown holding a wooden board above his head, ready to bring it down upon my head. What made him stop I do not know, but maybe it was the sheer terror in my eyes.

When I regained my composure I recognized the patient as being the one we had seen the previous night in the OR (operating room). Thus, that morning I learned my first lesson about the DTs (delirium tremens) and the long-term effect of chronic alcoholism.

Ruth A. Buzzard, Dawson Springs, February 23, 2012

CLINICAL TRAINING

During our clinical experience we were required to experience and learn about all major areas of medicine. This meant we spent three months in [each of] these areas: operating room, surgical unit, medical unit, obstetrics and newborn nursery, pediatrics, and a psychiatric hospital.

In addition, we spent a month each in the clinical lab, x-ray, and the diet kitchen.

I saw many clinical events not only as a learning experience but also as an opportunity to learn where I would like to specialize. When I was on OR rotation I loved it! There was so much to learn and I felt I did well in it. Most of the surgeons complimented me even though it is really hard to get a compliment from surgeons! There was only one drawback. The patients came in asleep and went out asleep. I liked personal interaction and I did not get it there.

Ruth A. Buzzard, Dawson Springs, February 23, 2012

OVERSIZED GLOVES

The first day I was in the operating room I scrubbed for a surgeon who was only about five foot and seven inches. He required a stool to stand on in order to reach the OR table. I am short and petite and needed a taller stool. In addition, the smallest pair of gloves they had was size seven.

As we worked the surgeon kept pulling my oversized gloves off my hands. He was patient and said not a word until he had completed the procedure. Then he turned to the OR supervisor and said, "I want size six gloves for this young lady tomorrow morning."

When I got there the next morning there was an ample supply of size six gloves!

Ruth A. Buzzard, Dawson Springs, February 23, 2012

RECOVERY FROM COMA

A young girl was admitted to the pediatric intensive care unit at UK medical center. I was the nurse on duty. She was comatose for a few days, but when she woke up she looked up at me and said, "Where did you get those Chinese eyes?"

I laughed and told her that I was born with them. Her question about my eyes were the first words she spoke after coming out of a coma.

Jo Ann M. Wever, Springfield, March 14, 2012

WEIRD HAPPENINGS

I remember two unusual patients during my early emergency room days, "Elvis's sister" and a stripper.

A patient claiming to be Elvis's sister came to the emergency room about 2:00 a.m. with her tape recorder, attempting to sing, dance, rolling on the floor, and making animal screeching noises. We placed her in a room near the nurses' station to observe her next show while trying to diagnose an "emergency" illness, to no avail. She promptly was assisted and discharged.

It definitely was a full-moon night when the next call came in due to a head and neck injury. A dancer/stripper was brought in from a local nightclub after falling off her pole on her head, claiming that the pole had been sabotaged. Actually, her pole had been greased!

Chesa Montgomery, Bowling Green, March 16, 2012

MOTOR VEHICLE ACCIDENT

When I received calls about this motor vehicle accident involving a sixteen-year-old boy my heart would skip a beat and I found it hard to breathe. I would run to the back of the EMS [emergency medical services] unit to make sure it was not my sixteen-year-old son.

I had been working feverishly that January night on this incident. I asked, "Did anyone find out what this kid's name is?" When they told me his name my legs became weak because he was one of my son's friends since they were toddlers. I fell against the supply Pyxis to brace myself.

He had started driving about eight weeks prior to the accident and was so full of life. That night his survival was not to be. I am so thankful I was there to hold his mother when the ventilator was turned off.

Chesa Montgomery, Bowling Green, March 16, 2012

FIVE TRAUMATIC EVENTS

It was "Black Friday" that morning when I arrived in the emergency room. Within twenty minutes trauma one arrived. It was a female found at home that morning and the paramedics performed CPR on arrival. Working code "A" was in progress but her down time had been too long. That wasn't how I wanted to start the day. Often how you start is how you finish!

I began her paperwork, calling the coroner, KODA [Kentucky Organ Donor Affiliates], [the] funeral home, her family, and so on.

Trauma two was called in over the emergency room radio. It was about a male who had been hunting with friends and fell over due to apparent AMI [acute myocardial infarction]. With all our efforts, there was still not any sign of reviving him. When someone's medical intervention is greater than ten minutes with a complete arrest the outcome is inevitable. The code was called and paperwork time began again. I thought [I was done], but not!

Trauma three began when I heard the paramedics on the radio tell about an older female involved in a motor vehicle accident and had major trauma. She arrived but was intubated, nonresponsive, had fractures and possible internal injuries. We began doing lab work, blood test, x-rays, and then called so as to transfer her to a level I trauma center. Upon arrival there was a hurry to get fluid boluses going, go to CT [a CAT scan], hang the blood, and try to stabilize her for the transport.

She never responded to me but I can still see her white hair that reminded me of my grandmother. Her outlook was grim but getting her to a higher level of care was her only hope. The flight crew arrived, giving me time to call a report and stack her chart with the others, then run to the restroom. When I rounded the corner I heard the radio call in for trauma number four. No! No! No! I thought, but only for a second, as there was the room to clean and restock just as I heard the gurney rolling through the back doors.

During trauma four I thought he looked familiar but you don't really have [time] to ponder personal thoughts. You have to keep focused to make every second of each patient's "golden hour," if even that. Trauma four was a CVA [cerebral vascular accident] or a stroke. So time is brain and you want to save as many cells as possible. So a test is run, CT, x-ray, fluids, medicine, and assess the patient for motor skills and rate any deterioration or progress.

I had the first line care started when one of the worst traumas was about to arrive, and that was trauma five. That trauma was about an eleven-year-old little girl with trauma from an MVA [motor vehicle accident]. She was thrown out through the sunroof of her family's van. They were traveling home after a holiday visit with extended family. All family members sustained injuries, from minimal to critical.

That was one time I could not move fast enough, assist in inserting chest tubes, get the blood going, more fluid boluses, start more IVs, try to wrap her scalp lacerations that were bleeding profusely on her blonde hair. I kept thinking faster, faster, faster, please move faster. As I was working on her head the emergency room medical doctor said, "Chesa, listen," as he lifted the stethoscope from her chest. I could tell from his expression things didn't look good. My body felt like lead as I placed the bell of my stethoscope on her little chest. Swoosh, with every chest compression, air, free air. She had a tear.

When I saw her father looking through the curtain I looked up at him to verify the diagnosis. I just nodded so he would not realize as of yet the nightmare words of every parent. The code was called and as I turned to go recheck trauma four, the emergency room doctor was sitting in the corner with his head in his hands. All I could do was put my hand on his shoulder and cry, but only for a minute as I had another critical patient that needed my help to not sustain lifelong disabilities.

He and his family were wonderful. They encouraged and helped me though I felt negligent in his interrupted care. I transported him to his room and wished him well. The next day I went up to visit him where he was recovering miraculously. I had recognized him correctly, a local businessman who did considerable charity work. I couldn't believe he was glad to see me, but he said, "I was hoping I would get to see you again. You had a bad day yesterday, didn't you?"

I said, "That's what I do."

Chesa Montgomery, Bowling Green, May 1, 2012

LEARNING FROM MISTAKES

As a labor and delivery nurse for over fifteen years I have made my share of mistakes, just as my nursing companions and doctors have done. Like most people, you seem to remember the first major mistake you made that could have endangered a patient's life. As nurses we are taught to care for people, not make things worse.

Working at Ephraim McDowell Regional Medical Center in Danville, Kentucky, I was one of the few registered nurses who could perform my duty on the birthing unit, including labor and delivery nurse, surgery circulating nurse, and surgery technical nurse. I enjoyed working the operating room both from the circulating viewpoint and the technical side, as they both had different challenges.

The largest mistake of my career happened when I was working as a circulating nurse. My patient was also a nurse at the hospital, the doctor was one of my favorites, and I had the best tech nurse in the world in my opinion. The surgery was an emergency cesarean due to a placental abruption, when the placenta tears away from the uterine wall. This is a scary situation under normal circumstances, but when you are operating on one of your own everyone is always a little on edge.

As the circulating nurse it was my job to keep all the notes and times for the surgery, give additional instruments or equipment to the doctor or tech, help the anesthesiologist with any requests, and count the lap pads [sponges] used during the surgery. I was basically a jack-of-all-trades, helping where I was needed the most, but my most important duty was making sure the sponge count was correct. Each lap pad is embedded with a thread that will enable it to show up on an x-ray if one is accidentally left in a patient, and this is where my mistake came in. I miscounted the sponges on one of our own nurses.

I had been carefully counting the sponges as they were thrown onto the floor by the doctor or tech, and I had them all neatly laid out in order for easy counting. At some point the tech dropped a sponge on the floor at her feet and I could not reach it, so I kept remembering to count the sponge under her foot. The problem was, at some point during the surgery she kicked the sponge out onto the floor and I did not realize it. I picked it up and added it to my pile as I continued to count the sponge I thought was still under her foot.

As we got to the end of the surgery I made one last sponge count before the doctor started to sew the patient up. I was still counting the sponge that was no longer under the tech's foot and because we had used more than the normal amount of pads I was sure we had them all. It was not until the doctor had finished placing the last staple in the patient's abdomen that I realized I was missing one sponge. When I went to get the sponge from under the tech it was not there. She told me she had kicked it out of the way so I looked everywhere for it, but my count continued to come out one less than what I should have had. To say the doctor and the anesthesiologist were upset is an understatement, and I was a nervous wreck!

When we were all totally sure the sponge was unaccounted for we had to have the X-ray Department bring up the portable x-ray machine to take a picture of the patient's abdomen. Well, sure enough, there was the sponge still in her abdominal cavity. With a few curse words and angry looks the doctor had to reopen the patient's incision and find the sponge. Luckily it was in the abdominal cavity and not the uterus so it was easy to retrieve.

I finally had an accurate sponge count and the doctor and tech resumed closing up the patient for the second time. I was humiliated because of the mistake I had made, and both of the doctors let me know exactly what they thought of me and my mistake. Naturally, I had to make out an incident report because it was an unusual circumstance with a patient.

When the patient woke up from her anesthesia I told her and her husband what had happened and instead of being mad at me she just laughed. "Leave it to me to have something go wrong. It's always the patients who are nurses that have had bad things happen." She was not upset, so that made me feel a little better.

I had to present my case to the incident reporting committee but nothing serious happened to me other than a reprimand. Believe me, though, after that night I always doubled and tripled my sponge counts before I let a doctor close up another patient. That mistake was a learning lesson for me because I never let it happen again.

Bobbi Dawn Rightmyer, Harrodsburg, June 5, 2012

DOCTOR'S IMPROPER ACTIVITIES

I was house supervisor with four years of nursing behind me when we received a call from the ED [emergency department] nurse stating I needed to come quickly to the ED and observe the physician and his treatment of the patients. Red flags immediately went up all over my radar. The nurse informed me the physician was unnecessarily exposing female patients. I thought that the nurse, being very modest, might have misinterpreted the physician's actions, so I accompanied him on his next examination of a female patient. She was about thirty-five years old and had a headache. He was going to listen to her lungs, so he pulled her gown down to her waist, exposing her breasts, and started to place his stethoscope on her chest.

I reached over and pulled her gown up to her shoulders. The patient looked at me with what seemed to be pleading eyes, and I remember her huge eyes. The physician looked at me and jerked her gown down again. I again reached across and gently pulled it up. After the third time of playing tug-of-war, the physician said he couldn't listen to her chest through her gown. Giving him the benefit of doubt, I told him he could listen to her chest from under her gown while I held it up. He then became angry and ordered me out into the hall so "we could talk."

I stopped him and took him into another room, closed the door, and asked him what he wanted to see me about. He blasted me for interfering with his examination. I let him finish with what he had to say but he overstepped his bounds when he stated he was the physician and I was "just a nurse." I replied that he may be a doctor and I may be "just a nurse" to him, but he would NEVER work in my emergency room again. I had the nurse tell all of his patients we had run into a situation and to please be patient while I called administration and the chief of staff and got another physician in there pronto. I told them about his actions toward the patients, the reflections it would have on the hospital, and the nurses were going to walk out if they did not immediately replace him.

Ten minutes later we had another emergency room physician in house working until another resident could be located. Small hospital, small town. Administration would come in every so many months and either tell me they had hired him back or would I give him a recommendation for work elsewhere. Very funny!

Jana Buckles, Lawrenceburg, June 9, 2012

YOU NEVER KNOW

Granny was accompanied by several family members when she arrived at the hospital. This was usual for the mountain people, who had to travel over one hundred miles to our regional medical center. Several hours had passed since Granny had fallen on her way up the creek, a hundred slippery steps from the home place to the barn.

The situation and the family activities were not unusual for the time and the place. They had been sent to our center because the local doctor had felt Granny's injuries warranted x-rays and a medical specialist. The family was concerned and protective as well as a bit in awe of the city, hospital, and the staff. They had waited patiently while Granny was examined and reexamined as our corps of physicians went through their paces, prodding, nodding, consulting, x-raying, and making final decisions. Finally it was deemed that Granny had broken her pelvis when she fell. Treatment for this particular type of fracture was to send her home, give her pain medication, and for her to walk as much as she normally would.

The family did not question what they had been told because they had brought her to the specialists and were prepared to follow instructions. They accepted that they had to drive back to the mountains, taking

Granny with them. And though they were tired and worried they were sure they had gotten the best medical care for Granny.

Part of my job as a nurse in the emergency center was to assist patients in getting into their cars and make sure they were safely on their way. It was a clear, cold night and still very dark in the parking lot as I helped make Granny comfortable in the back of the old mud-splattered station wagon. They had plenty of blankets and I "loaned" them a pillow or two as we made ready for their departure.

At last everybody was loaded into the wagon and we had discussed the way to the interstate, so I asked a final question, "Do you have any more questions before you leave?" I was confident that the doctors and I had covered all bases, so I was taken [a]back when Granny's son, the driver, said, "We-1-1-1, I'm not sure how we'll get Granny across the swangin' bridge."

Nothing in my urban nursing classes had prepared me for dealing with getting an old woman with a fractured pelvis across a swinging bridge at any time, let alone in the dark during the middle of the night. So I asked, "Why do you have to get across the bridge?" The son said, "The doctor told us to take Granny home and her home is across the swangin' bridge."

Having walked, or I should say, having teetered across a few swinging bridges in the past, I was able to visualize a scene of the family trying to hold on to the rope and Granny while creeping there, swinging and swaying, as the boardwalk screeched and rebelled. I knew it would be a nightmare. However, the family felt they had to follow the doctor's instructions to the letter, and if Granny was to go home, then home was where they planned to take her. With the concreteness of the unsophisticated and innocent, they were prepared to do the nearly impossible. I thought for a bit and then announced that I had the authority to allow them to take Granny to someone else's home, one that was on this side of the bridge.

The family talked things over and decided that Granny could stay with her daughter and not have to be carried across the bridge. I agreed that this was a good plan and suggested that they get started home.

The taillights faded as I watched the overloaded wagon pull out of the parking lot and head down the ramp. I thought about how carefully our instructions must be given, but most of all I acknowledged the importance of a nurse being prepared to deal with "swangin' bridges" of any sort.

Jeri R. White, Lexington, June 16, 2012

MR. NEW OVERALLS

The emergency room had quieted down. So far it had been a fairly normal Friday night—victims of auto accidents, shootings, children with runny noses, women in labor, a couple of men with stabs and slashes, some with heart attacks and other common complaints had all been treated and sent on their way.

I looked up as I heard clothing rustling and feet shuffling. I had seen a lot of people in my years as an emergency room nurse but I had never seen anything like him before. The elderly man standing before me was pink and shiny. His gray hair was combed as a small boy combs his, still damp and parted ruler straight. His white shirt was buttoned to the top and his blue overalls were still like new. I couldn't keep from smiling but I noticed that no one was with him and he obviously was not seriously hurt or ill. I asked how I could help him, so I thought I had heard and seen it all but I had no experience to fall back on when I heard his answer. My first thought was that I had not heard correctly. I decided that if I asked more questions and listened very carefully I would grasp what this was all about.

He said, "Lady, I want to turn myself in."

He said that very clearly and seriously. Still not being able to deal with what I had been told, I asked another question: "Are you sick or hurt?"

He stated that he was not sick and was not hurt, then said again, "I just want to turn myself in."

My mind was busy trying to find a category to fit his puzzle into, but he didn't fit anywhere. Obviously he had been able to care for himself and had no observable behaviors that appeared paranormal or in any way psychotic. He seemed very certain that he wanted to turn himself in so I had more questions to ask him before I could ever guess what was needed. My first question was, "Would you like a cup of coffee?" I knew that I had to sit down, and having a cup of coffee might make me think more clearly.

I told the staff I would be busy for a while and to let me know if they needed anything. Mr. New Overalls, as I had mentally dubbed him, took our coffee into the office and sat down. I knew this was going to have to be taken one step at a time and very slowly. I was grateful that it had gotten quiet and I had the luxury of time.

He began his story slowly and carefully, so I prompted him along from time to time. Here is what he told me: "I ran away from the hospital twenty-three years ago and I am tired of hidin' and runnin'. I can't stand it no more." He shifted his chair, sipped his coffee, and continued: "I was in the insane asylum in Indiana and didn't like it much, so one day I just walked away. They had put me in that place and I just didn't like it, so I left and just walked on away and kept on going." He looked at me so as to make sure I was listening to what he was saying.

He stared out the window as he continued his story, then said, "I would work on a farm since I grew up on a farm and was a good worker. I'd work a few weeks or sometimes a few months and then move on to another farm, sometimes in Kentucky and other times in Indiana or Ohio. I never had trouble findin' work. I kept to myself though, so didn't get to know people and didn't let 'em know me. It was hard and lonesome not talkin' and I was afraid to talk to them. I can't write and was scared to anyway, so I never kep in touch with my kin because I was afraid they would turn me in. Lady, I just got tired and can't do it no more." He turned slightly and looked at me with watery eyes, then asked me, "Can you help me?"

I sat there very still, with my thoughts jumping around, seeking ideas for helping him and then how hard his life must have been with years and years with no family or friends. The idea was unbearable to me since I was close with all my family, often seeing and talking to them. Helping Mr. New Overalls turn himself in was going to be a challenge, and I was sure that I would have to be creative. I had some ideas but was pretty sure the system would not run smoothly.

Mr. Overalls actually did make it back to Indiana. The on-call social worker for the emergency room arranged for him to have temporary housing at the Salvation Army Lodge downtown, provided a cab to take him there, and made arrangements with the Indiana hospital for him to have transportation to get there.

The last I heard about him was that he had been released from the hospital and had moved back to his hometown. He had found work on a farm in that area and was getting some help in his efforts to locate his only brother who had moved away after his parents had died.

Jeri R. White, Lexington, June 16, 2012

SERVICE IN EMERGENCY ROOM

I worked in a hospital emergency room in my hometown during some summers while I was in nursing school. The nurse that was in charge on night shift was sort of in charge of the whole hospital, which had only about thirty-five beds in it. With other nurses taking care of the patients you could do a rotation. So if somebody came into the emergency room I would usually go with that nurse to see what I could do.

In that small town most of the emergencies were people who got drunk from nine to five, persons that had got drunk and had automobile accidents, or maybe a child that had taken too much aspirin and needed to have their stomach pumped out. So because of that experience, I didn't care to take care of drunks who came in cussing, fussing, and carrying on; thus I decided the emergency room was not for me. So I never chose that as an area to work in. Typically, I later worked in surgery.

Told by Martha Hill, Glendale, to Mark Brown, June 30, 2012;
provided by Kentucky Historical Society, Frankfort

NEED FOR AN EMERGENCY ROOM

One day a man was brought to the floor on a stretcher, screaming with pain. Of course, all the other patients and their families were within eye and ear distance. The gentleman had had hot tar accidentally poured on him as he drove down a road where new paving was being put down. It was a freak accident. He had his arm stuck out the car window, giving a left-turn signal.

I recall treating him before he was transferred to Cincinnati. Back then the emergency room was not open during the day. It wasn't needed, since the hospital staff members were there.

It seems simple, doesn't it?

Evelyn Pearl Anderson, London, July 18, 2012

YOU CAN STOP FAKING NOW

There is one thing guaranteed when you work the midnight shift in a busy emergency room, and what it is will be drama. Until you have lived it you can't imagine what lengths someone will go to in order to convince the ER staff that they are sicker than the person who just signed in ahead of them, or the histrionics used in order to impress, or manipulate, their significant other person.

I was working triage one night when a group of eight or ten young people, probably in the age range of eighteen to twenty-two[, came in].

Most of them were male but a few females were in the group. They were very excited, and all of them were trying to tell me what was ailing their friend. The friend was wobbling up to the triage desk in a gait that appeared unsteady. He had one hand holding his head and the other hand clinging tightly to one of the young ladies in the group.

Just as he reached the desk he suddenly fell to the floor but was being very careful not to land too hard. After he fell he started "flopping" around, doing his best imitation of one having a seizure. Pardon me if I sound cynical; it is because I am. An untrained eye may be taken in, but anyone with even limited experience in the emergency room cannot be fooled by a fake seizure.

Of course, he suddenly became the center of attention of all his friends, not to mention everyone else in the waiting room. I wasn't worried about the patient at this point due to the fact [that] my main concern was crowd control. His friends were becoming very loud with a bit of hysteria mixed in, and the other bystanders were beginning to gather around. I knew we had to get him into the ER just as soon as possible.

An orderly quickly brought a gurney, and he along with a security guard helped me load the still-flopping patient onto it. I knew that once we got through the double doors leading to the main treatment area the doors would lock and the mood in the waiting room would quiet down.

Once we were through the doors and I heard the sound of the lock securing them, I bent over the young man and said, "Okay, jackass, you can quit faking now because your friends can't see you now."

Wow, I know of no medicine that could stop seizure activity better than that short sentence! Immediately the patient sprang from the bed and attacked me. He was almost instantly restrained by security, but not in time to keep the tunic of my uniform [from being] literally torn off of me, and two large scratches across down the front of my chest.

I was able to get a scrub top to take the place of my tunic, and the doctor insisted that I get a tetanus shot because of the scratches. Otherwise, I was fine.

Oh, by the way, final diagnosis for the patient was "intoxicated and stupid."

Ah, now you can visualize the drama in an emergency room.

George W. Williams, London, September 21, 2012

I Feel Like I'm Gonna Go

I suspect that every nurse had that one incident way back in the beginning of their career that they would prefer to forget. Only problem is, their cohorts won't allow that. I am not sure if it was my rookie year, but it was certainly early in my ER career during which I had one of those moments. Until the day I left Mary Washington Hospital I was never allowed to forget it.

It all started just as the midnight shift was ending, about 6:00 a.m., when the rescue squad brought in a very obese forty-seven-year-old male complaining of crushing chest pain, some difficulty breathing, pale and sweating. This man was the very picture of a myocardial infarction, the classic heart attack.

Perhaps because of my relative[ly] limited experience I was more or less acting as the "go-fer" ("Go fer this. Go fer that.") while the more seasoned nurses took on the more critical tasks in what was a life-threatening situation. Because the patient was showing signs of congestive heart failure the doctor ordered that IV diuretics be given, then turned to me and told me to place a catheter into his bladder to evaluate the fluid.

Even though the patient was in a great deal of distress and probably did not even hear me, I carefully explained the procedure to him as I would to any patient. I set up the sterile equipment that I would need and began to perform the procedure. As I started inserting the catheter I told him that as the catheter passed the prostate gland he might feel some discomfort but that it would be over in a second or two. Passing the catheter by the prostate gland will often stimulate the need to urinate.

Just as I felt the resistance as the catheter made contact with the prostate, the patient said, "It feels like I'm gonna go," to which I responded, "That's okay, that's what we want you to do."

The words were barely out of my mouth when the patient went rigid, jaws clenched; alarms sounded, the cardiac monitor showed ventricular fibrillation, soon followed by a flat line. We were unsuccessful in reviving the patient, but even in a somber setting the tears in the nurses' eyes were due to laughing at me, the "new nurse."

I remember one nurse saying, "George, you know the last words that guy heard was, 'Go ahead, that's what we want you to do.'"

Even though I later became the nurse that most of the doctors wanted with them when treating a cardiac patient, I never lived that day down.

George W. Williams, London, September 21, 2012

A FRIEND IN TIME OF NEED

The summer of 1989 was much the same as any other summer at Mary Washington Hospital in Fredericksburg, Virginia. The emergency room area was too small, much too busy, and desperately understaffed. I had just recently been assigned as charge nurse on the graveyard shift even though I was in truth less experienced than several of the nurses that I was now assigned to supervise. Making the situation worse was the fact [that] I had planned to travel to Georgetown, Kentucky, the last week in July to attend our family reunion. This had become a virtual ritual with me for the last weekend in July, and I did it every year.

However, this year the staffing situation was near critical; it needed life support. As the weekend for the family reunion grew closer it became obvious there was no way I could leave. I had not missed a reunion in years, but I felt the obligation to stay and help manage the ER. I knew there were some who resented the fact that I had been selected to be charge nurse, and I did not want to give them any reason to fan the flame. Also, [I was] staying to make sure staffing was adequate because it was part of my DNA. So come Friday night, I was clocking in to work instead of driving to Kentucky.

Well, at least it appeared that we might actually get off easier than usual tonight. Midnight came and the triage area did not have its usual line waiting to sign in. About 1:00 a.m. the rescue squad radio sounded the alarm. The Stafford County EMT [emergency medical technician] service advised us they were on the scene of a one-car accident where the driver was dead at the scene. At the hospital we referred to this event as code gray. The squad needed a doctor to officially end life-saving efforts and declare the victim dead. At that time we instructed the squad to go directly to the morgue and to bring the paperwork to the ER for charting purposes.

When the EMT brought the paperwork in I glanced at it and my heart sank. The name written on the top line was the nineteen-year-old son of an old and dear friend. What could I do now? Nothing. The body had already been taken to the morgue at a local funeral home. It was 2:00 a.m. by now and business was picking up as the bars closed, so I did my charting and resolved that I would contact my friend in the morning. Although we had been very close at one time, we actually had not been in contact for a year or so. I knew they [the boy's parents] had separated at one time, but did not know if they had reconciled.

About 2:00 a.m. the registration clerk called and told me that "the mother of the code gray is in the waiting room." Oh God, what do I do now? I did not think I was ready to deal with this yet, but I walked to the waiting room. Immediately upon seeing me, she threw herself into my arms, crying hysterically. I held her and kept repeating, "It will be okay."

Then I realized that the man with her was not the husband/father, so I did not know him. Maybe she saw the question in my expression because she gathered herself long enough to introduce him as a friend.

I asked about her husband and she said, "We can't locate him." He worked at one of the large airports outside Washington D.C., located about an hour away. She said she had called but they could not locate him, but they took a message to call immediately.

I told her I would try to locate him, then called the airport police, identified myself, and asked if they would locate the father and have him call me immediately. They said they would do it. It was about fifteen minutes when he returned my call and told me instinctively that something was very wrong. His first words were, "Was it C—— (the son), or B—— (the mother)?"

I told him the son had been involved in a very bad accident, trying not to be more specific over the phone. But he pressed me, saying he needed to know how bad it was before he began the one-hour drive down I-95.

I will never forget the long, loud wail that came over the phone. I had just told a close friend that his only son was dead at the age of nineteen. I then called my wife, got her out of bed, and asked her to come to the ER to be with the mother, as I still had other patients to see to.

The next few days and weeks were very difficult. The mother was totally inconsolable. The one thing I took from the experience was that I had been there for friends when they needed me most. Both parents told me over and over how they sincerely believed that God had caused me to miss my family reunion in order for me to be there for them at that time. They told me it meant so much for me to be there rather than having to deal with a total stranger.

God does indeed work in mysterious ways.

George W. Williams, London, September 21, 2012

Nurse Known as "Bumphead"

We had one patient with poliomyelitis who was in an iron lung. He was Bobby Wayne [last name omitted] from the mountains of southeast Kentucky. He was a fragile, sweet little six-year-old boy. It was an experience caring for Bobby Wayne in an iron lung. We were happy to care for the little guy. He seemed to like Maxine and me especially. He named me "Bumphead." I don't know why, but that was my name according to Bobby Wayne.

I was working the eleven-to-seven night shift, in fact, several nights straight. After I had administered all the medications and any ordered treatments, I would be in the nurses' station charting before the end of the shift. I would hear this sweet little voice coming down the hall, saying, "Bumphead, hey Bumphead, daylite's a-comin'!" He spoke with his wonderful mountain accent.

One night worm medicine was ordered for Bobby. He was so frail and ate poorly. Well, I will tell you that the worm medicine really worked. Goodness! What a sight, and in an iron lung! The little fellow was sure to have felt better. This is the way it was; the student nurse in charge was also the one to clean up the worms from his body, bed, and floor. That was okay because it helped the little guy.

Seemingly, "Hey Bumphead, daylite's a-comin' outside" became a wake-up call. Someone came from the *Lexington Herald* to do a story about Bobby Wayne. The newsperson took his picture. He was very proud. There were not many people still living on a totally iron lung. The newspaper sent or brought eight to ten copies of Bobby Wayne's [picture]. He gave Maxine and me a copy of the picture.

Seven-year-old Michael, who suffered from leukemia, was also there. He was down the hall. Michael and his parents lived in northeast Kentucky. His aunt had been a high school teacher of mine, so he was very special to me. As Michael's condition worsened, his parents stayed in the room or nearby. His mother was expecting a new baby in a few months. I could be in the room caring for Michael in the early morning hours. We would hear, "Bumphead, hey Bumphead, daylite's a-comin' outside!" Michael's family would smile and say "Bumphead" very kindly.

On New Year's Day of 1961 Michael died. It was very sad for all of us. It was always a sad, humbling experience to be with someone at death. A child's death was especially sobering. The priest came to offer the last rites and to comfort the family.

Evelyn Pearl Anderson, London; reprinted from Anderson,
Daylite's A-Comin' *(Baltimore: Publish America, 2007), 77–78*

LOCAL HAILSTORM

In 1998 we had a major hailstorm when I was on duty. We were asked for volunteers to go to the emergency room to help with the injured when they came in. One gentleman came in with a laceration that needed suturing.

When asked what happened, he said that while driving down the street it started hailing and busted the windshield, so he had to try to drive looking out the side window, but as a result he got pelted in the head.

Times like that were truly dangerous.

Jenny Burton, Bowling Green, May 8, 2013

3

BABY BIRTHS

Whether it happens at home, in a neighbor's house, or in a hospital—which were constructed somewhat late in certain parts of Kentucky—the arrival of a precious infant is typically a joyful event. Every now and then mothers-to-be prefer not to talk to nurses, doctors, and even family members, due perhaps to the pain they anticipate having during the birth process. Some mothers resist support from nurses or doctors. Nonetheless, the birth of a baby is often very much a family affair, with family members and friends present to celebrate the baby's arrival. Not often does the first sight of a new baby cause the father to faint, as recounted in the first story.

Today most childbirths occur in hospitals, but numerous grandparents and great-grandparents across the Commonwealth have wonderful memories of the times when babies were born at home or in a neighbor's house, with the assistance of midwives or other women. Many of the stories in this chapter describe the work of midwives, who help the mother both before and after the birth.

Although nurses encountered certain dangerous events, such as a mother unknowingly smothering a new infant while the two were sleeping together, most found that mothers and fathers typically did all they could do to help the growth of their precious infant.

VIEWING NEW BABY

This is an incident that occurred while I was working in the OB [Obstetrics] Department at Hopkins County Hospital in Madisonville, Kentucky. Some of my fellow nurses and I were sitting at the nurses' station doing our charting after a busy evening at work. Suddenly we heard a loud noise from down the hall and also a big commotion.

As we looked down the hall we discovered that a new father who had been looking at his new baby through the nursery window had passed out cold and fallen onto the floor. He'd made it through labor and delivery, and I suppose by this time the reality of it all had sunk in and it was just too much for him.

Charlene Vaught, Portland, TN, August 2, 2011

STILL WONDERING

After forty-three years I still wonder about this pregnant woman whose circumstances haunt me and I yearn for answers that I know I will never get. Who was she? Where did she live? What circumstances led her to hide her pregnancy? What events led her to face alone the birth of her baby in a strange town and then to give her baby to a local adoption agency? How lonely did she feel? What burden of guilt did she carry through life, or did she?

She was a well-groomed, well-spoken, brown-haired white female in her mid- to late twenties and was from an unknown place just "out of town." She moved to Henderson two weeks prior to the birth, and from all accounts, according to local persons, she lived alone in an apartment and spoke to no one, not even via telephone, except during her appointments with the gynecologist. We, the nurses on the obstetrics ward, intuitively participated in the silence so as to validate the unspoken acknowledgment of her shame. We dared not to ask her any questions. We told each other that her choice spared her harsh labels that would be a lifelong burden never forgotten, not only for her but also for her child. In local Kentucky culture, the child as well as the mother bore the shame [of an unwed pregnancy] throughout life.

Her eyes were sad, she never talked so as to express her feelings, and we did not and could not ask. We assumed this was not something she wanted to do but something she had to do. Any debate was long past and she was yielding to her task. Each of us asked if we would and could serve as counselor.

During her birth labor she moved cooperatively but silently. She showed very little emotion during the birth, not even expressions of pain. After the birth there were a few hours when she was considering seeing and holding her baby, but those handling the adoption counseled [her] not to do so. It would only make matters worse, so she didn't see her baby.

The mother signed the papers and left, as she had come to us, alone. The task was done, or was it? All of us nurses felt empty. We had denied the joy of birth that fed our love for our work. We wanted to take her in our arms and help her mourn. We wanted to tell her we cared and that we knew her pain. We wanted to tell her we supported every choice she made. We wanted to talk, but this took place in 1968 in a small southwestern Kentucky town, and an unyielding culture closed our lips and made us participants be silent.

After forty-three years I still wonder if it is unfinished business, unwillingly accepted.

Dr. Kay T. Roberts, Louisville, December 19, 2011

The Itchy Problem

After working as a registered nurse in labor and delivery for many years you learn rather quickly that weather can affect [the] number of patients you may see in the course of [a] one-night shift. Old wives' tales say women will start labor with the change of the moon, but as nurses we know that a change in the barometric pressure will bring out any number of patient complaints.

One night in particular I was working with my operating room scrub technician and we had a revolving door going through the birthing center. We had only one woman in actual labor, but the rest of them had a range of urinary tract infections to Braxton Hicks contractions to preterm labor. There were three birthing rooms and a two-bed triage room. All the beds were full and here came another patient.

The emergency room also had every stretcher in use, so we did not know what to do with the new patient. The scrub tech said, "What about the on-call bed?"

The on-call bed is where the doctors would sleep when they were actually in the building. There was one for the males and one for the females. Because one of the male doctors was watching on the baby to be born our only choice of beds was the female on-call bed. Big mistake!

The patient was only twenty-four weeks and complaining of low-back pain. After checking fetal heart tones and doing an admission assessment, we obtained a urine sample to be tested for a urinary tract infection, the most common cause of low-back pain in early to mid-pregnancy. We obtained the catheterized specimen, and as we did that we were horrified to see lice in the patient's lower region. Upon closer inspection, lice [were] also found in her hair and in the hair of her husband. We had put a patient with lice into the female on-call bed; thus we would never live this one down.

Needless to say, both husband and wife were treated for the lice infection and we had the housekeeping team sanitize the female on-call room. We ended up feeling itchy for the rest of the night!

Bobbi Dawn Rightmyer, Harrodsburg, February 22, 2012

CHRISTMAS BABY

As a mother of three children it is hard working on the holidays. Nurses do not get holidays off, so on Christmas Eve 1999 I was watching the clock, waiting for the time to pass so I could get home before my children woke up. I was a labor and delivery nurse, and although I had seen a few patients throughout the night no one was in active labor.

Just as the clock turned six o'clock, one hour before I could leave, a man came running through the birthing center pushing his girlfriend in a wheelchair. "It's coming," he yelled. I rolled my eyes because normally when a man yells, "It's coming," there is usually nothing to worry about. Forty weeks is considered a full term, so when I found out the patient was only twenty-seven weeks pregnant I assumed she had a urinary tract infection or some other simple ailment. You know what is said when you assume something.

Getting the patient in the triage room, I quickly found the fetal heart rate and reassured the parents the baby was fine. So far the patient had not said a word, but as she started to moan, I noticed how hard her abdomen was getting. She was having contractions. When I made my cervical exam, I found the patient to be eight centimeters dilated, when ten centimeters is full dilatation. With a twenty-seven-week baby I was afraid of an imminent delivery, so I called the doctor to the triage room. I was lucky enough to have the on-call doctor in the hospital, and he came immediately to the triage room.

Within three minutes of the doctor examining the patient the tiny baby was born on the stretcher of the triage room. He was so small he fit in the palm of my hands. I had just enough time to warn the nursery before the baby was born, so I wrapped the baby in a blanket and dashed to the nursery and the waiting warmer. This baby was a fighter, because he let out a little cry.

Drying him off, we began to secure an airway and start intravenous fluids, and the pediatrician was a few minutes away. The baby was so fragile you could see his veins through his paper-thin skin. The obstetrician came into the nursery to see if he could help. He had left the patient with the operating room scrub technician. We called the University of Kentucky Hospital to inform them we needed a transplant [transfer] to a level-three neonatal nursery since our hospital was only a level two.

When the pediatrician arrived he took over working on the baby with my assistance while the nursery nurse prepared the paperwork for the transport. In those minutes after the delivery I forgot all about time. All I could think about was this Christmas miracle lying before me. I couldn't turn away from the teeny living soul fighting so hard to live. I stayed at the hospital until the UK Neonatal Team arrived to pick up the baby. I watched, fascinated, as the team worked to stabilize the baby for transport.

That Christmas morning it was after nine o'clock before I got home. All the way home I bemoaned the fact I had missed the grand opening of Christmas presents by my three children. I knew my husband would take loads of pictures, but it would not be the same as actually being there. I tried to tell myself there would be other Christmases, but I couldn't get this Christmas out of my mind.

What a surprise when I arrived home and found my three children and my husband patiently waiting for me on the couch in front of the Christmas tree. They had opened no packages. My family had delayed Christmas until I got home. After unwrapping all the presents and cleaning up the mess I told my family about the Christmas miracle baby as they listened in awed fascination.

Bobbi Dawn Rightmyer, Harrodsburg, February 22, 2012

UNFORGETTABLE BABY BIRTH

No matter how long they have been working, every nurse has one patient that is hard to forget. Be it good or bad, some patients are truly unforgettable. My patient came in the form of a redheaded fifteen-year-old girl who was in labor with her first baby.

Granted, this was a situation where a "baby" was literally having her own baby, and I really felt sorry for the little girl. But after a few hours of her childish behavior my sympathy and empathy had flown out the window.

When this patient first arrived she had her entire family with her—parents, siblings, aunts, uncles, and even a few cousins. They were not happy to be sent to the waiting room, but we needed some room in which to work and there were just too many people there. The patient was obviously in pain but my fellow nurse and I were having a hard time getting her in the bed so that I could do an examination. Mothers-to-be often had pain, but after nurse's support some also requested to be examined. Some mothers were stubborn when offered helpful assistance by nurses.

When I finally convinced her to lie down I found she was in active labor, so we started admission procedures. The patient demanded she wanted no epidural for pain. Epidurals are becoming a standard of pain management for most women in active labor and are very efficient for relaxing patients and making the labor process more enjoyable. Epidurals are also easier on the nurse because the patient is not in much pain and is able to cooperate more in the birthing process. I could tell by this girl's attitude that we were going to have problems if she did not receive an epidural.

With each contraction this girl would scream to the top of her lungs and cry for her mother. At first this did make me feel a little sorry for her, but whenever I would try to help her she would cuss me out with words that would embarrass a sailor! When this would happen I no longer felt sorry for her. She would refuse to be examined, so it was difficult to see how her labor was progressing. In addition to cussing at me she began to kick at me with her legs, and one time I got close enough that she grabbed my ponytail and almost yanked my head off!

We tried numerous times to get her mother to try to calm her down. The mother kept repeating, "I don't know where she learned those words because she doesn't use them at home." I still do not believe that is true. Even with active labor, if the patient had not used these words in the past she would not suddenly start using them.

When the ob-gyn entered the room it took me, another nurse, and the girl's mother to hold her down for the examination. The doctor went ahead and broke her water, which made it easier for us to keep track of the fetal heart rate. He told the girl we would call for an epidural and she then screamed "NO" at the top of her lungs. "I don't want that huge needle in my back."

No matter how hard we tried to offer the epidural, the more stubborn and out of control she got. I was able to give her some pain medications through her intravenous line, but it would only last a few minutes and then she would be screaming again.

That might not have been so bad, but I had another patient in labor and she was a nervous wreck listening to the little girl scream. My second patient already had her epidural and was feeling very comfortable, but her nice, quiet birthing experience was being ruined by the antics of the fifteen-year-old girl.

When the girl was finally close to delivery the doctor came to check her again, and again we had to hold her down. She was completely dilated, and when the doctor told her to push she again screamed "NO!," then kicked the doctor in the head. To say he was a little less than pleased is an understatement. He tried to get the girl to push but she refused. We continued trying to get her to push, all the while watching the fetal heart rate on the monitor. She kept up her screaming and flatly refused to help.

I was so fed up that I told the doctor to leave the room and I turned to her family and told them, "If you don't calm her down and get her to push we're going to be here all night. We are going to be sitting at the desk until the baby is crowning." I then turned and left the room.

The doctor and I sat at the desk, which was directly across the room from this little girl, keeping our eyes on the fetal heart rate monitor to see how the baby was tolerating labor. The doctor was so mad, and I tried to calm him down but I was angry myself, so I did not have much luck.

Finally the mother came to the door and yelled at us, "It's coming, the baby is coming!" I got up first and went to the room, and just as I was spreading her legs to check her cervix I saw the head crowning. The doctor was right behind me and as I managed to get the girl into the stirrups and break the bed apart, the doctor was preparing for delivery.

The delivery went much smoother than the labor and she had a healthy baby boy. As the doctor cut the cord and handed the baby to me he began numbing her bottom up because she had a huge tear that needed to be repaired. By the time the placenta was out this girl had calmed down and couldn't feel any of the stitch work the doctor was doing.

Almost like Dr. Jekyll and Mr. Hyde, this girl's demeanor changed right before our eyes. No longer cussing and screaming, she was asking for her baby, and as I handed [her] the little bundle she cradled him in her arms. I was surprised when she started to cry again but I realized these were tears of joy.

Although I have never had another patient like her, she is one that I will never be able to forget. I was physically and emotionally drained and the doctor looked worse than I did. As we proceeded on to check our other patient we both looked at each other and burst out in laughter. The doctor said, "Just another night in labor and delivery."

All I could do was nod my head and laugh.

Bobbi Dawn Rightmyer, Harrodsburg, May 18, 2012

BABY BIRTHS AT HOME

When I was doing midwifery service [in the Frontier Nursing area] a mother-to-be would come along and ask for my service when they were expecting the baby's birth. I think they more or less had a baby each year. We gave the mother very, very comprehensive antenatal care. . . . And they got specimens taken of feces and blood and smears, then had their measurements taken, their blood pressure checked, and all the things we could do for antenatal care. But it was very regular and very thorough.

Actually, the mother-to-be came in once a month for the first three months until they were seven months pregnant, and then twice a month following that, then during the last month it would be every week or more often if necessary. The babies were always born at home. The hospital was always called and the husband would come to get the midwife. For the baby's delivery it might be twenty-four hours before the baby arrived.

These husbands and wives were well schooled into what they should do, so everything was ready when we got there. A baby's birth was very much a family thing, so I think everyone was there.

When it was all over we got on our horse, loaded with saddlebags, and went back to the hospital or home.

Told by Lydia Thompson to Carol Crowe-Carraco, 1978;
provided by the Louie B. Nunn Center for Oral History,
University of Kentucky Libraries, Lexington

FEAR OF RISING RIVER LEVEL

There was this girl that was expecting her first baby and I remember that she had just had a bit of disproportion because she understood the terms but her head hadn't been [thinking] during the last week. I was very anxious because the river was rising and there was no way of getting her to the hospital. However, I decided that she ought to be in the hospital just in case she had to have a cesarean section. We went all the way around by the backwoods, and when we finally got to the hospital there had been so much rain the road was flooded out. Well, she got out of the jeep and walked up the steps. She was so quick and agile, she got up the steps and then got into the hospital and the baby was delivered before I got my body up there [chuckle].

Told by Lydia Thompson to Carol Crowe-Carraco, 1978;
provided by the Louie B. Nunn Center for Oral History,
University of Kentucky Libraries, Lexington

The Role of Midwives

Because the midwife has a background of assessment skills we learned in our first term, were are able to assess the pregnancy and to know what is normal and what is abnormal. As long as the pregnancy is normal the midwife can diagnose and take care of the woman until the baby is born and even thereafter. Many midwifery services are set up in that perhaps the woman only sees a midwife throughout the whole process if she remains normal. Here at Frontier Nursing Service it's a little bit different because we have a physician right at hand, and she sees the patients as well. But we're completely trained in all the prenatal care; we're trained to follow a woman through labor, to do the delivery, to give the postpartum care, and to take care of mother and child up until their six weeks after delivery, and then assisting the mother in choosing family planning methods and helping her to find follow-up care for the child. I think the difference in midwives and MDs is that here again we have the background of nursing, which is all the teaching and the counseling and emotional support that we can give to a patient, which we feel is a priority in midwifery.

I think when people read about natural childbirth, and there's a lot of books written about it now, they have the concept that natural childbirth is going through the whole experience without any medication, no shots, no anesthesia. As midwives we're trained to realize that there's a time and place for both injections and for anesthesia. We feel that a woman should be awake and cooperative, because by [her] being awake and helping in the birth process the baby has a safer delivery. In other words, the baby is not under the influence of a lot of anesthesia. Or, as in the past, you know, when a mother is given anesthesia often the physician has to use forceps to pull the baby out, where we midwives are very strong in believing that if we can help the mother maintain her control, she can push the baby out and it's much easier and much better for the health of the child.

We also believe that our sustaining presence is a method of giving help to cope with the pain. And we try to be with our patients almost constantly through labor, depending on how much they need us, and that includes all supportive care, or just being aware of where the mother is at. But we do use pain medications that assist the mother to cope, but they do not take away her control. That way she is still aware and she still is able to do what she wants to do and what she needs to do to have a safe delivery. If a mother has had preparation by doing a lot of reading and if she has [in] her own mind determined to go all the way without medication we stand by that decision. We try to use our sustaining presence to accomplish that goal. But often I will tell the mother that we believe in natural childbirth but with some medication if it is needed.

There's so many different areas that we try to teach a woman who is pregnant about, getting her to understand her own body and what her body is going through, how it's adjusting to the pregnancy, and how the pregnancy is affecting the way she feels. And this takes in all the way from her social interaction with her family, her sexual life, mentally and physically of course. As a whole, at Frontier Nursing Service we have a teaching list that probably has 150 items that come under these different areas that we try to talk about and try to pinpoint problems. If someone comes in to us at two and a half months, which is about ten weeks of pregnancy, then we like to see them every month after that until their seventh month, and then it's every two weeks, and then finally during their last month it's once a week. So we see someone very often and we're able to carry out this teaching as we go along.

I think women have a lot of fear about what they're going through, so by touching on different topics we're able to isolate what those fears are and educate her. . . . Perhaps it is not quite as valuable for couples to go to these midwives' classes as it might be with an MD. One difference between a midwife and an MD is that a midwife will take at least twenty minutes per visit, whereas an MD might take only five or ten minutes.

If the husband comes in the clinic he is included in everything, such as examinations and all discussions, because we like to have the family unit rather than just the mother. However, his presence depends on the couple. I think basically the difference is in the teaching in the whole concept that a pregnancy creates a change not only in the woman but within the family structure, as they'll have to prepare for the next child.

Told by Karen Slabaugh to Dale Deaton, March 23, 1979;
provided by the Louie B. Nunn Center for Oral History,
University of Kentucky Libraries, Lexington

Birth Control

Back then there were a number of individuals who felt it wrong, reli-giously wrong, to have anything to do with birth control. However, there were still quite a few that would. So they became acceptable [accepting] as they got to know a little bit more about what it really meant. There were always certain individuals, aside from certain other individuals, who really needed to stop having families because they have had very difficult pregnancies [but] that, because of their husband or because of the church, didn't feel they could do anything about it. And we would spend hours talking with them trying to convince them that it was all right. Sometimes it worked and sometimes it didn't. We did some tubal ligations, but they were few. It's only in more recent years that it has become acceptable to have a tubal. Because that was a big step; it was permanent and you really had to be sure. And even though you may have had enough children with this present man, if something happened to him you might want to have a family with another man.

And if they weren't willing to have a tubal, people back then lived day to day. If they were pregnant they didn't worry about that child or that pregnancy until the child had arrived. They wouldn't think about picking out a name beforehand, getting clothes ready, or maybe making a bed. Truly, most of them didn't because they slept with their babies. That used to worry me because I had a couple of mothers with their first child who rolled over on their babies and smothered them. But that was an exception, as most of the mothers did sleep with their babies. I tried to get them to not sleep with their babies, but they did it for warmth. They also did it because of the rats. There were also stories about snakes coming into the houses and sucking on the baby's bottle and things of that sort. So mothers were afraid to leave the child in a separate bed.

Told by Elsie Maier to Dale Deaton, December 5, 1978;
provided by the Louie B. Nunn Center for Oral History,
University of Kentucky Libraries, Lexington

Babies Born at Home

There were a lot of home visitation follow-ups. For instance, we had a tremendous number of home deliveries when I came here [during the midfifties] and you really had to know how to work in the homes because we had a radius of three miles, and if people were delivered at home inside of three miles we had to visit them every day for ten days. There were family homes that [sheltered] the whole family, which included the mothers, fathers, and grandparents, with whom many of them lived in those days. I think there were something like three hundred families for each nurse, but that's a wild guess. So there were about six hundred families for us two nurses within a three-mile radius. . . . You didn't have to take the outside people, thus you didn't have to accept them if you didn't think you could manage that amount of work . . . , but I don't think we ever did turn people down. However, many of them didn't come to us if they were going to be referred somewhere else.

The thing is that they really came to the hospital . . . if they were outside that far and they couldn't be reached by us because we didn't feel we could take them. If we couldn't reach them they came into either our hospital or another one to be delivered. In my day at the hospital there were people who were well on in their babies' coming, [with]in twelve to fourteen days, but they were still staying at home because they chose to refuse the hospital. In the early sixties some of them did have their sixteenth baby at home.

There's one person I know who lives on Rockhouse and she was a young woman who was employed as an aide in our hospital and she had her first baby at home. She's had her second baby at home, and I can't remember if she's had a third baby or not. I do know that she's never been in the hospital to deliver her baby, but she chose it that way. She has always been normal, so it has been accepted.

Told by Molly Lee to Eliza Culp, February 6, 1979;
provided by the Louie B. Nunn Center for Oral History,
University of Kentucky Libraries, Lexington

A QUICK BABY BIRTH

One afternoon I was working in the labor and delivery area when at the change of shift a Hispanic lady comes in with her male friend, obviously very pregnant. She was speaking no English and also understood very little English also. Lucky me, I was the only one who happened to speak enough Spanish to get by, and the only words she knew at that time were, "Baby come." Needless to say I understood what she meant! No physician in house, the ED [emergency department] physician was too far away, and the baby was crowning.

I yelled for a tech that was still in orientation, but she was the only one in view, and [I] told the lady to push, and out slid the infant, which breathed and cried. The tech lady said, "Congratulations, new baby boy," to them in Spanish. I finished up what I had to do and then called the physician. Of course, the physician did not say "good job," he said, "Why didn't you call me? How long has she been there, and why didn't you check her when she arrived?"

As most physicians do, he spoke before he got the whole story. Once he found out she had been there less than three minutes prior [to] delivery he changed his tune! So chalk up one for the nurses!

Jana Buckles, Lawrenceburg, June 6, 2012

CARING FOR NEW BABIES

Mary Breckinridge always came around the hospital when she came over. Of course, she was always interested in seeing the mothers and babies. She was horrified when she found out we were getting the mothers up a little earlier than she was accustomed to. But we were getting very busy and we had very few beds. And it was a question of getting the mothers ready in case we had to discharge them early to make room for other mothers. But she would say to me, "Brownie, I really don't mind you getting them out of bed if you would just make them walk on all fours. Nature didn't intend man to stand up so soon."

But we did have to get them up and get them out fairly soon. Of course, it's proven that it's satisfactory, but we had to be very selective because I agreed with her that these mothers probably got the only rest they had when they came in to have a baby.

So we tried to keep them in bed a bit longer. And the mothers having their babies had to take care of their baby when she got home.

The older girls in the family were taught to take on needs and to learn very quickly how to do them, such as how to make cornbread. And they always learned how to bring wood and water.

Told by Helen E. Browne to Carol Crowe-Carraco, March 26, 1979;
provided by the Louie B. Nunn Center for Oral History,
University of Kentucky Libraries, Lexington

UNUSUAL BABY BIRTH

When a nurse works in labor and deliver[y] long enough you see things that will stick in your mind and you won't forget, especially if it turns into a lawsuit later. I was responsible for an obese pregnant woman and tried most of the day getting her into labor with Pitocin, which requires fifteen-minute interventions the entire time until delivery. We like to call obese women "fluffy," a much nicer term, don't you think? Anyway, this patient thought she could not move while she was in the bed and had the Pitocin running in her IV. No matter what I told her, I tugged and pulled on her all day long until I was frankly exhausted by the time she went into good labor.

Having no monitor, a laboring patient, and the unborn child is a very hard job [in] which one must be prepared to recognize and treat signs of fetal distress appropriately. After pulling and tugging on her and talking until I was blue in the face, I was sitting in front of the labor monitor documenting on her chart and watching the fetal heart rate pattern and the contraction pattern. All of a sudden her contraction pattern had gone haywire and I rushed into the room thinking she was adjusting the monitor straps herself (a nurse never knows what a patient is going to do next) and found her standing beside the bed by herself. She said she got tired of being in the bed and climbed out over the side rails to stand up for a few minutes. I told her to get back in bed and practically had to force her back into the bed. Finally I reminded her in a pleasant way that she had made me push and pull on her all day, and now she figured she could move by herself since she walked in on her own this morning but I didn't think she could.

I got her back to bed and then called the physician, who came over to see her since she was as frustrated with her antics as I was. The physician decided she needed a cesarean if she had not had the baby by a specific time. This specified time came and went and the physician told me to prep her for surgery. Since she had internal monitors on, they were taken off and the patient draped in the usual fashion. I assisted the physician during the cesarean. Once the skin into abdominal incision was made, we immediately knew something was not right. I swear I saw a little hand stick out but the physician said it was a foot. No matter, since the infant came flying out of her abdomen to the pediatrician, with the physician yelling, "Intra-abdominal pregnancy, intra-abdominal pregnancy."

The physician looked at me, stating that did not sound right. We both started laughing afterward, since we both knew this was incorrect; the infant had been where it was supposed to be until the incision was made, and evidently the uterus tore for some unexplained reason, making it look like the infant had developed in her abdomen. The infant and her mother were both fine and made a speedy recovery.

The physicians and nurse were a bit excited for the rest of the day.

Jana Buckles, Lawrenceburg, June 9, 2012

THANKS FROM BABY'S MOTHER

While serving as a midwife, if there were two midwife nurses there the father of the forthcoming child would stay outside or go into another room, but the father always helped if only one midwife was there. I love having a father there to help me because this is their child too.

This is not about a father, but after I had graduated from midwife school I had to go to a woman up a creek to help deliver her baby. She was one-legged and she had been seen by a physician. She did have extra bleeding and I was very annoyed with the physician because he had sent me back to deliver her baby. She did have extra bleeding and I got all set up to go in and do removal of the afterbirth when it came loose and came down. So you not only knew your patient very well but you and God knew each other quite well too.

After it was all over the mother said, "I knew you were scared, but I also knew you'd do it."

Believe me, that sort of faith does something to you.

Told by Grace Reeder to Carol Crowe-Carraco, January 25, 1979;
provided by the Louie B. Nunn Center for Oral History,
University of Kentucky Libraries, Lexington

CONFUSING TRAVEL TO DELIVER BABIES

We almost always went on house calls by ourselves, because while two nurses lived on a district together usually we each had somebody else due, and if I got a call out the other nurse would not dare go because she had some [patient] due, and if they came for her they would wonder where she was. She wasn't home and I wasn't there either, so we had to be available for a call. If we were both not on call, occasionally we would go together, but almost always we went alone.

An interesting thing was that we had telephones at the district centers and a few families and local stores had telephones, but the telephone operator locked up the place and went home about four or five o'clock every afternoon, so there was no telephone at night. Since most babies seemed to arrive at night, we would hear scrunching of gravels as a car stopped down on the road and the running feet of the father coming up steps to the clinic building. If you weren't fairly fast on your feet there would be the jangling of the cowbell that hung outside the door. I don't think anybody ever jangled a cowbell on me because when I was on call and I knew there was another nurse there, I slept with one eye open and always heard the vehicle stop, and as I already had my housecoat on I was at the door by the time the person ran to the door.

I have occasionally been sort of sleepwalking and found myself driving at high speed down the road in the jeep with my saddlebags for delivery and wondered, "Just where is it I am going?" If there were headlights in front of me it was okay because I knew that was the man who came to get me, so I would follow him home.

If there were no taillights I did have to pull over to stop and think about it for a while.

Told by Jean Fee to Rebecca Adkins Fletcher, June 15, 2002;
provided by the Louie B. Nunn Center for Oral History,
University of Kentucky Libraries, Lexington

SERVICE IN ISOLATED AREA

My friend and I were the nurses that gave immunization shots, and we did the baby once monthly at the clinics that we would hold either in our center or in out-clinics. Different people would either donate the use of their living room or bedroom, or in some cases we had an extra small building that was in some farther out part of our district that may have been a little more convenient since not everybody had a car. And if they did have a car, Daddy was probably at work. So Mama and the kids were walking.

It seemed reasonable to have families closer to where people were. It was not realistic to expect people to come for miles and miles. If somebody had to go miles and miles it was us, because we had transportation and many times they didn't.

I remember being at a clinic when a lady came riding a mule across the creek and up to the clinic and then came in and said she'd come to register up. When we checked her she was about seven months pregnant, and we didn't even see her again until she called while she was in labor. She lived at a place that took the nurse over an hour to get there while driving a jeep.

Told by Jean Fee to Rebecca Adkins Fletcher, June 15, 2002;
provided by the Louie B. Nunn Center for Oral History,
University of Kentucky Libraries, Lexington

BABY SURVIVES BLEEDING MOTHER

I got a telephone call after Christmas from a woman who was bleeding and she didn't even know whether she was pregnant [again], as she had a fairly young baby, and that meant that birth control, that was used by a good number of women who were breast-feeding, doesn't work for everybody, so I determined that this woman was six or seven months pregnant and she was bleeding and that's a no-no. She was bleeding rather severely, but the only way to get her out was across that river, and the river was up and my jeep was drowned in the middle of it. Her husband's car was parked in my yard for the same reason, that he couldn't get it across the river. Well, I made calls up there morning and night to check on her. She wasn't in labor, just bleeding.

She was sent to bed rest, which is very difficult when you have several small kids. However, her husband proved to be much more co-operative than many, and she did pretty well [on] bed rest but she kept losing blood. I had a little hemoglobin meter and I went up there one day to find that her hemoglobin was reading seven on my meter, not ten, which was considered okay. I said to her, "We've got to go. That's all there is to it, we've got to go."

By this time I've got my jeep out of the river and it was functional once again. I told her that I would come in the next morning when frost and mud won't be deep on the road. However, I went to see her that evening and she was bleeding more vigorously, so we just had to go. So I went to get my jeep and eased it up the hill on the road that was just barely wide enough for the jeep. We got the woman on board, and her husband and I started back down the hill to cross the river but I knew we weren't going to cross that river with that many people in it, so her husband walked around by the bridge and we got through the river.

We loaded her in her husband's car and took off for Hazard, where I had called a doctor I knew to tell him about the problem. He had more or less had a hemorrhage over the phone about it, and he said, "Oh, I'll meet you there."

I said, "Hold it. I've got at least an hour of jeep work before I can hit the road, and then three-fourths of an hour on the road."

Oh my God! Believe it or not, he was already there when we got there. He then did an immediate C-section, got a live baby, which I did not expect, and the baby had an unusual blood type, and the lab tech that came in and checked the blood was a match for it. I think the Lord was truly looking out for that girl.

Told by Jean Fee to Rebecca Adkins Fletcher, June 15, 2002;
provided by the Louie B. Nunn Center for Oral History,
University of Kentucky Libraries, Lexington

CHILDBIRTH ON THE MOUNTAIN

A lady was pregnant, and one month before she had her baby she and her family moved about five miles from here, where it was over the hill and down the hill. In January 1947 [?] the father came for me in the morning. Two other nurses had already gone out to see her but lost track of the woman after she had moved over the mountain. So the father came to get a midwife but the midwife wasn't there. I went with him and we walked. There was nineteen inches of snow, the worst snow I had seen here in the mountains. I was afraid to take out my horse because there was a lot of [ice in the] creek bed and I was afraid my horse might cut his feet on the ice. It's very treacherous to take a horse in a frozen creek. So the father, who was carrying the bag, and I walked up the hill, and then we walked down the hill.

When we got to his house his wife had already had the baby, so all I did was clean up. But there was nothing in that home, I mean nothing. There was just one crust of bread and one pot of coffee and we all shared it. Then, after I'd cleaned up the woman, I looked at the man and said, "Now you had this baby, so you get something for the family to eat. I don't care whether you beg, borrow, or steal, you've got to get them something to eat. They're your family and your responsibility."

I think I was a little mad and a little hungry, too. I was also tired, having walked all that distance when they could have stayed there. I couldn't understand them moving away up into those mountains, but I'm sure they had their reasons. The father walked back down the mountain with me and carried my saddlebag all the way. I said, "Now I'll carry the saddlebag so you can go back and take care of your wife, and I mean take care of her and see that she gets something to eat because she needs it."

That's the only time I ever talked so sternly to anybody. Of course

I reported it to the social worker, but what could be done during winter when it is that icy and cold and you have nothing to go by. Anyway, I carried that saddlebag the rest of the way and I was so tired. All I could say was I knew what it was like to be an automaton pulling one foot in front of the other. It was rugged during the early days, so what could you do?

I don't know that I did my best but I did the best I could do at the time. I must admit I didn't go out for a couple of days after that, as I wasn't able to!

Told by Gertrude Isaacs to Dale Deaton, November 15, 1978;
provided by the Louie B. Nunn Center for Oral History,
University of Kentucky Libraries, Lexington

CHILDREN'S FAVORITE HOME

At times a child is born before the marriage of parents and very often the child has found a home with its grandparents. Sometimes the child went back to parents, sometimes it did not. When I came back here in 1969 I was interviewing a lady with her children and I asked her about her family, how many children she had. At that time she had three children with her but the oldest child was not with her, so I asked her, "Well, where is he?"

She said, "Well, my grandma helped me with him while he was a little boy and he was so much happier with her that we never took him back. So he is more like her child than mine. But he is still my child and if anything should happen to her I would take him back."

Up here on the hill there's a fellow that lives there and his grandchild lives with him. The child's mother had a divorce, so he went to live with his grandparents. I think there's much more shifting of children in this way. I'm not sure whether or not they think of it as "our child" more than "my child" and "your child."

A lot of things I don't know, but if I could go back and work with the people in their homes I would dearly love it, but I haven't got the strength these days. That's why I go around town once in a while and stop in at every little place to chat with them awhile.

Where else can you go in a business place and stop to chat while you find out all that's going on in the community?

Told by Gertrude Isaacs to Dale Deaton, November 15, 1978;
provided by the Louie B. Nunn Center for Oral History,
University of Kentucky Libraries, Lexington

BEFORE AND AFTER BIRTH

[Prior to the availability of hospitals] all the babies had to be delivered at home, and that was all right with us because we had special delivery bags for them. We had this bag in which we carried all supplies that we would need for delivery. These bags were to be used only for the delivery itself. In our general bags we carried an emergency kit in case we got caught somewhere, and the mother was in labor. . . . As soon as we came back from the delivery we had to empty those bags completely.

We fixed the baby up and had to stay an hour and one-half after delivery to make sure that everything was all right because you might be five miles away from home. If you had just rushed off as soon as the baby was born, anything could happen. We saw the mother and baby for the first ten days and did all the things that we could do. Then we saw them once weekly for the first month, and then every month for the first year. . . . We also took care of the whole family as well as the mother, and we kept very careful records of it. We then followed the baby's first year and then followed them as toddlers and then through school. Twice a year we saw them when they were in school. I mean, we soon were what you'd call family nurses as well as midwives then.

Of course we had to write up the record of the delivery, exactly what happened and all about the birth.

Told by Betty Lester, Hyden, to Jonathan Freid, March 3, 1978;
provided by the Louie B. Nunn Center for Oral History,
University of Kentucky Libraries, Lexington

SAD STORY, HAPPY ENDING

There's one baby birth event that stands out in my mind. As midwives we weren't supposed to go outside the five-mile limit. We weren't supposed to go a step beyond that. Well, I was at Bull Creek one Thursday and this woman came in to register and I asked her all the various questions. Then I asked her where she lived and she told me she lived over on Big Creek. Then I said, "Oh my goodness, I can't take you there. You'll have to come into the hospital to have your baby."

She quickly said, "I can't go to the hospital," and I said again, "I'm sorry but I can't come because it's about seven miles."

Tears came into her eyes; then I looked at her and asked, "What's the matter?"

She said, "Well, I've had one baby and my baby was born dead, and I want a baby very badly, and if you'll come and look after her, I'll have that baby."

Well, what could I do? I simply couldn't do anything. Well, tears came into my eyes, too, because she wanted that baby so badly and she had enough faith in the nurses to feel that her baby would be born alive.

I said to her, "Well, if you'll come to the clinic every time I want you to and do everything I want you to do I may be able to take you home."

Her eyes brightened up at that and she said, "I'll come," and then I told her, "I will come over to see where you live because I want to see if you have everything there that I need."

When Mrs. Breckinridge found out what I had promised, she said to me, "Betty, you cannot leave your own patients; you cannot neglect your own patients for an outsider. If you'll promise me that you won't neglect your own work to go over there you can go because you can ride. You've got a good horse, so you can do it, but don't neglect your own work."

Of course I told her I wouldn't even dream of it, then said, "If you'll let me go just for the delivery and just for the postpartum, if she comes to me for her prenatals, will it be all right?"

She said yes, so I did go. The woman's husband came for me in the middle of the night and we had all seven miles to ride. When we got there she was in labor but took a long time, and if she'd had a local midwife I don't think she'd have had a live baby because it was a very difficult delivery and I did have a hard time. I sweat blood getting the baby, and I got a live baby so it was worth it.

The baby was a girl, and she grew up, got married, and I saw her when she was pregnant. So I went and she was going to have her baby in the hospital. So I went to the people in the hospital and said, "May I come into the delivery room when she has her baby?"

"Well, you can take the baby if you want to."

I said, "Well, thank you very much," and did the delivery. So, she had a live baby boy.

Well, the baby boy grew up, got married, and that shows how old I am. His wife was going to have a baby, and they saw me again. I said, "Well, I'm not going to do anything about it this time but I will be in the delivery room." Then I went to the supervisors and said, "Please, may I observe this delivery?"

They said yes, so I sat in the back of the room and watched it. So, I'm a great-grandmother!

That's my outstanding story. There have been other ones, but that's the one I truly treasure.

Told by Betty Lester, Hyden, to Jonathan Freid, March 3, 1978;
provided by the Louie B. Nunn Center for Oral History,
University of Kentucky Libraries, Lexington

LABORS RELATED TO CHILDBIRTH

Nurses had certain obligations, but I'm not familiar with requirements, as they fulfilled the obligations of the frontier nurse to the people in the community. For instance, in cases where babies came there was a five-dollar fee charged for delivery. However, included in that service were specific obligations that the nurses had to require. In other words, the nurse would then require that the mother come into the clinic, or she would stop and see the mother at certain intervals, maybe once a month for the first three months, and maybe twice a month, then maybe once a week as the time grew nigh.

Then, after the delivery of the baby came the postpartum care of the mother and the care of the child. But it wasn't just, you only go when you are needed, there was a definite schedule that you were supposed to perform as you worked with each one of those families.

Told by Dorothy Caldwell, Burlington, to Marion Barrett,
January 19, 1979; provided by the Louie B. Nunn Center for
Oral History, University of Kentucky Libraries, Lexington

DELIVERIES THEN AND NOW

We have a lot to do in order to make home deliveries of babies safe. I think we need to institute the system they have in England, where they still have some home deliveries, but they are less over there. The Flying Squad, which is a team back in the hospital, will rush out to whoever is providing home delivery, and this includes the obstetrician, blood, a midwife, and lab technicians, and they rush out to the home. But it can be safe only if you have careful prenatal care so that you know the mother that is going to be at risk is brought to the hospital. Careful prenatal care is the reason for the success of the Frontier Nursing Service. Watching out for the abnormality in time for medical intervention helps to prevent it from becoming a crisis. It is essential to make every effort to get the woman at risk into the hospital. And if the woman absolutely refused, we then made every effort to get two midwives on the case. That's what the midwifery supervisor used to do a great deal of in early days; that is, go to be with the midwife when she went to a case at risk.

There's a great change in the training of the nurse-midwife at the present time, especially compared with thirty or forty years ago. I think the change is a real challenge. When we first started the school here in 1939, childbirth was considered a normal course of events in the life of a woman. With the explosion of medical technology it has been extremely difficult for the young student midwife to consider childbirth as a normal course of events. That is because she is faced with all the horrors that can happen to this woman. As a result, when this woman comes in, certainly into the teaching situation like the Hyden Clinic, although I used to scream about it all the time, I am convinced that the first thing students learn to do is to look at the reports that come back, and she's learning. So these are significant, and she's going to talk in front of the patient. We aren't explaining to the patient what this really means, so we convey apprehension to the mother. I'm sure we introduce this and I'm sure we increase apprehension. Back when it was a simple affair and we didn't have all these tools to work with . . . everything went along perfectly normally.

However, you do have to have a very astute midwife to watch out for abnormalities. She listened very carefully to the mother, who didn't really know [that] if she had a headache that it was significant. You had to be very careful to listen, to ask questions, and to draw this out, because the headache, to the midwife, could be a very important symptom, but not necessarily to the mother, because she might have thought this was just the normal course of events. So you had to be a good interviewer and listen very carefully to what she had to tell you and then assess it very carefully. Today it's an altogether different kind of issue.

Childbirth is not the normal course of events it used to be anywhere in the developed countries. I think this is why the public is revolting. Women are fed up with all this sophistication. There are centers now, I'm glad to see, where they say it certainly isn't necessary to use the fetal monitor on every mother. So they are interfering before they really need to. We don't know before they got this fetal monitor if every normal newborn didn't have a change of heartbeat as the labor went along. But now the first time it starts to drop they immediately interfere. Meddle-some midwifery is something we were always warned against. I used to say that in this service the biggest danger is hemorrhage; anything else could wait, provided you had a well-trained midwife taking care of the case.

If the labor is being long and forceps might be indicated, provided the midwife knows ahead of time so the mother doesn't get too exhausted, it can wait. You have time to get to the hospital. But for hemorrhage you have to intervene, and you never can forecast hemorrhage.

Told by Helen E. Browne, Wendover, to Dale Deaton,
March 27, 1979; provided by the Louie B. Nunn Center
for Oral History, University of Kentucky Libraries, Lexington

Initial Disagreement between Nurse and Doctor

I recall the time I was working in the hospital in Berea and this lady who was a roster patient and had no doctor came in and was admitted to the Labor and Delivery Unit. So the roster patients were assigned to the doctor who was on call when they came in for delivery. One night when I was working a roster patient came in and was admitted to the L & D Unit and the next doctor on the list was one I knew fairly well, who liked to play cards. I think when I called him to tell him that a patient was there I interrupted his card game!

He wasn't very happy but he came in and proceeded to check the patient and said that she's not ready to deliver yet. Well, I thought she was. So he went into the doctor's dressing room and proceeds to change into scrubs. The patient had a contraction and I thought the baby would be delivered right then and I would be responsible for delivering it. So I just hollered out to him and said, "You'd better get in here because the patient is about ready to deliver."

So he came in and found out that she was about ready to deliver, so he proceeded to slowly get ready for delivery, and he was mumbling things to me. Finally I said, "If you're talking to me and want me to do something you're going to have to speak up so that I can understand you."

He looked at me and said, "I would just like for you to get out of here."

I said, "Well, somebody has to take care of this patient, so I'm going to stay."

Well, he got the patient delivered and got her into the recovery area and the baby was okay. The next day the doctor came in and said, "I want to apologize to you. You were right last night and I was wrong."

I said, "Thank you, I know that's the case," or something like that. We were friends forever after that and he always came when I called him! But that one time sticks out in my memory.

Told by Martha Hill, Glendale, to Mark Brown, June 30, 2012;
provided by the Kentucky Historical Society, Frankfort

UNEXPLAINED PREGNANCY

It was at the Oneida Mountain Hospital where I heard that women came to the hospital saying they were in "the family way," which meant the baby was about to deliver. The work wasn't hard there. As is said in present times, there was a lot of down time.

I do recall one woman who came in declaring she had never "known a man." Her obvious late-stage pregnancy made that statement pretty much a mystery!

Evelyn Pearl Anderson, London, July 18, 2012

BIRTH OF TWINS

I assisted Dr. Robertson with baby births at the George Dimmit Memorial Hospital, Humansville, Missouri. Twins were born late one night and both procedures were done in the same room on the top, third, floor of the hospital. It was a large single room in the center of the building with skylights all around. The large elevator screeched to the second and third floors. The elevator door would open and you had to pull an accordion-type door to enter or exit. It was quite interesting to transport a patient up and down in the elevator.

Dr. Robertson permitted the grandmother-to-be to come up to the delivery room. The patient's husband was a trucker and on his way home from Kansas. As soon as the first baby was born there appeared to be another baby still in utero. I said to Dr. Robertson, "I believe there is another one," to which he responded, "I don't think so." But as he was checking, sure enough, the other baby began to come.

By this time the grandmother was so excited that she ran out the door and then down the steps to the first floor to tell her husband. It wasn't long until both of them were back in the delivery room to view the two little boys. Dr. Robertson was as happy and proud as they were.

Evelyn Pearl Anderson, London, July 18, 2012

The Hospital Didn't Name the Baby

A lady delivered a beautiful baby girl at an area hospital without any complications. When she was ready for discharge and the hospital was inquiring regarding the baby's name to be placed on the birth certificate, she stated that the hospital had already named the baby.

When questioned further, she stated that the baby's name was on the bassinet. The person completing the birth certificate was confused and told the mother that the hospital did not name the baby, that this was her decision. She adamantly told the person that they did name the baby and her name was Female, pronounced Fee Mah Lee, which is how she pronounced the name.

Now the hospital only puts "baby girl" or "baby boy" on the card in the nursery bassinet.

Janet Smith, Irvine, January 14, 2013

Baby's Birth Not Anticipated by Doctor

Before all the monitoring, nurses would sit by the bedside of mothers in labor. We watched their progress, checked dilatation, observed when they moved through the stages of labor. On this particular day there was a mother who had several children already and was progressing nicely through her labor. I believed she was about ready to move to the delivery room.

I called the doctor, who was in the doctor's lounge waiting for the call. He came in to check her and reported she was not ready. I replied when she pushed, [indicating] she is imminent.

He replied, "Not yet," and then walked out of the room, but then she had another contraction and there was the baby. I was not going to say, "I told you so!"

Patricia A. Slater, Petersburg, March 6, 2013

Near Death of a Baby

A younger lady followed this older lady, who was her mother, into the emergency room. A quick telephone call was made to the physician on call. The young woman was admitted to the hospital while the baby was placed into a rarely used incubator. Soon we realized the woman had not yet passed her afterbirth. She was cared for, and the baby miraculously lived for three days.

Evelyn Pearl Anderson, London, March 27, 2013

Premature Birth

A few years ago when the emergency doorbell rang at this small rural hospital, I was the only RN [registered nurse] on duty. A nurse's aide and I went downstairs to open the door when an older woman walked in and flung a dishtowel in my arms, then said, "Here." Being quite surprised, I looked carefully into the terrycloth contents and found a very, very premature baby!

Evelyn Pearl Anderson, London, March 27, 2013

Comments, Not Stories

In the delivery room with family members at the bedside, a boy was delivered and one of the family members asked if he was circumcised!

A new mother was trying to decide what to name their baby girl, and she said [that] Virginia "sounded like noise."

A newborn in the nursery was being prepared for circumcision when the permit was signed by the mother, who asked if she could have the foreskin. However, she didn't have a reason.

When getting a patient ready for delivery we noticed she had an earring in her labia, which had to be removed. After delivery, the mother went to the bathroom and expelled a large item; on feeling and seeing it she said, "What was that?"

    On examining it they found out that it is to be three four-by-fours [sponges], folded and placed in the vagina after delivery. That was left in place when it shouldn't have been.

Jenny Burton, Bowling Green, May 8, 2013

STILLBIRTH

I was working in our local emergency department one night when a nurse from the triage section wheeled a young lady back who was screaming in pain. The complaint the lady checked in with was sharp abdominal pains. She was screaming, so the triage nurse brought her on back to be worked on. There was a team of nurses getting the lady out of the wheelchair onto the bed. As we moved her she kept screaming and crying.

The lady probably weighed three hundred pounds easily. The nurse that checked her in was asking her all about her medical history while others were working on getting her undressed, blood work, IV started, etc. As the patient was lying there we had to get a urine [sample], and the only way that was happening was to get the specimen through a catheter. So we got the lady in position for the catheter as a nurse calls out, "I see a head!" Well, we were all in shock because this lady was having a baby. Quickly we called the OB doctor and yelled for the emergency room doctor, STAT!

This young lady didn't even know she was pregnant. People were running everywhere trying to get the tools we needed to deliver. This was an ER, not a labor and delivery unit. This event was something you would only see on TV. The ER doctors were working so diligently to have a speedy, successful delivery. EMS was there to help as well.

All of a sudden the ER doctor told her to push. After a few pushes the baby's head was out. As I looked, the baby's head was very deformed. The ER doctor tried to suction the baby but couldn't get any movement. After the mom delivered the baby it was already blue. The team immediately jumped in and started CPR. It was too late, as the baby was stillborn.

As we researched the situation, of course the woman had no prenatal care. The doctor said the baby was about thirty-five weeks old and had been dead for about five weeks.

These are stories we never want to encounter as nurses, but sometimes we don't have a choice.

Dana Burnam, Bowling Green, July 29, 2013

4

Humorous Accounts

Readers may not laugh at all of the stories below, but the nurses re-counted them with a great deal of humor. There is virtually nothing to add to that. Some of the stories focus on doctors, sometimes as they wondered what a patient was trying to explain, while others involve nurses' and patients' responses to doctor's pranks.

Doctor's Laughter

During a particular day at the Hopkins County Hospital in Madison-ville, I was gowned and gloved in my sterile dress and was setting up one of the tables in the delivery suite. We were not to touch the tables, so I was attempting to drop one of the bulb syringes onto the sterile table. As I dropped it, it bounced off the table, and when I got another syringe it did the same thing.

One of the doctors was seated out in the hallway and was appar-ently amazed by the whole scene because he was laughing and shaking his head. Well, I finally was able to get another syringe on the table.

Charlene Vaught, Portland, TN, August 2, 2011

Misunderstood

Strange things happened when I was working the midnight shift at nursing homes back when I was still a nurse's aide, and this happened at Gowan Nursing Home in Robinson, Illinois. One night an old man was keeping the whole facility awake by shouting loudly, "I need an enemy. I need an enemy."

I tried several times to calm him down, but to no avail. Frustrated, I told the other nurse's aide, "If he keeps on yelling like that, he's going to have a lot of enemies." We eventually figured out what he wanted was an enema.

Charlene Vaught, Portland, TN, August 2, 2011

PRANKING STOPPED

One of our residents had a jolly ol' time finding the nurse's aide's sweaters hanging on the wall railings. He would sneakily tie the sweater sleeves in knots and then wait for the owner's reaction.

One night one of the girls decided to reverse the prank, so she tied his trouser legs in knots. When he tried to put them on he became quite angry.

Apparently the joke wasn't so funny when the tables were turned on him!

Charlene Vaught, Portland, TN, August 2, 2011

SURGEON DROVE TOO FAST

This surgeon I worked with in the OR was a character in more than one way. He performed surgical operations in two different hospitals separated about thirty miles apart. One morning, as usual, he was speeding down the highway from one hospital to the other when a policeman pulled him over and gave him a ticket.

The doctor paid the officer twice the amount and said, "I'll be back in about two hours going the same rate of speed."

Boy, that's quite a story!

Ruth A. Buzzard, Dawson Springs, February 23, 2012

SEARCHING FOR SITZ POWDER

An experienced nursing student told me to look for the Sitz powder. I was a student nurse in my first clinical rotation. I looked everywhere that I thought it might be and some places where it could not possibly be. When I told her I could not find it she gave me a stern look and walked away.

I was sad and embarrassed that I had failed to find the Sitz powder. Later on I was told there was no such thing as Sitz powder!

Jo Ann M. Wever, Springfield, March 14, 2012

IDENTIFICATION OF A THREE-H ENEMA

My first job after graduation was on a medical-surgical floor with patients who had a variety of diagnoses. Many had x-rays that required enemas until clear. The 11:00 p.m. to 7:00 a.m. shift, fondly called the night shift, had the responsibility for this task. I was thankful I did not work the night shift.

On occasion the secretary in x-ray would call and say that the patient had not been prepared well and needed a three-H enema. One day when she called, suspecting that she did not know what the three-H enema was and that the radiologist had told her what to say, I asked her. Just as I suspected, she did not know what it was. I proceeded to tell her that a three-H enema was "high," "hot," and a "hell" of a lot.

I tried not to laugh when there was a long silence on the other end of the line!

Jo Ann M. Wever, Springfield, March 14, 2012

DOCTOR REFUSES LIGHTS

I walked into a room that was only lit by sunlight. I asked the neurosurgical physician who was examining one of the babies if he wanted me to turn on the light.

He said no, because he had been operating in the dark for years, so why change now?!!

Jo Ann M. Wever, Springfield, March 14, 2012

REMEMBERING HOW TO SAY THINGS

I used to say to Mrs. Breckinridge, "Sometimes I get lost and I can't remember where I was."

"Never worry, child," she said, "I've done that so many times. All you have to do is look at your audience and say, 'Now, where was I?' Someone may be willing enough to say something; otherwise it jerks your own mind back as to where you were."

Told by Helen E. Browne to Carol Crowe-Carraco, March 16, 1979;
provided by the Louie B. Nunn Center for Oral History,
University of Kentucky Libraries, Lexington

NAKED ELDERLY WOMAN PATIENT

There is always the one about the "sundowners," a term often used to describe older patients who after the sun sets turn from Dr. Jekyll into Mr. Hyde. One particular night when the moon was full I was working in the emergency room of a small hospital. The staffing was one nurse, one resident, and one unit clerk. We saw thirty patients each shift after office hours and on weekends and holidays. These were all types of patients with all kinds of complaints.

I was busy trying to take care of everything at once and keep the physician on course. If you did not keep the physicians busy they would scuttle off and hide or watch television; then you would have to play "Find the Doc." I kept hearing water running somewhere in the emergency room but was unable to locate it. Busy as we were, time went by and the noise continued on and off. Since the patients' doors were shut most all of the time for patient privacy, standing and listening to sounds at each door was highly overrated. I was hearing the water again as I passed the trauma room, threw open the door, and there, standing in the hopper in the room, was a ninety-year-old female, naked as a jaybird, doing a dance in the water as it splashed all over the floor. My mouth fell open and she said, "Well, don't just stand there, child, bring me them thar clothes you've got on. I've gotta get this wash done before them menfolks gets home and wants dinner."

Just when you think you have heard it all!

Jana Buckles, Lawrenceburg, June 9, 2012

OLD MEN NOT WANTED

I can remember a little ol' lady, and I'll never forget her. She was long since past the childbearing stage, but as you took the oral history she said, "You know, I've been bred twenty-one times, and this will be the first time any man other than my husband has ever seen me."

The fact that she was "bred" stuck in my mind, and she was very honest about it. She was very, very shy. She carried her money in a belt that fitted underneath her clothes around her waist. She also had a pouch, [a] little pocket, so this is where she kept her money. And since the doctor was going to do an abdominal as well as a pelvic, this had to come off. She was very reticent about this. I persuaded her that we could take it off and pin it around her neck so that she would have it on her body all the time, and that was quite all right with her. But I had to be right there because she wasn't so sure she wanted any old man to examine her, even if he was a doctor!

Told by Grace Reeder to Carol Crowe-Carraco, January 25, 1979;
provided by the Louie B. Nunn Center for Oral History,
University of Kentucky Libraries, Lexington

Travel Directions Needed

Mrs. Mary Breckinridge and I, along with a nurse I think was Jean, were traveling around. Having never been in the mountains very much, I was really intrigued. What I'm about to tell was so typical of Mrs. Breckinridge. After driving all around I was goggle-eyed, since I hadn't been around in the mountains at that time. But I knew that nurses were expected to travel from one center to another. Finally I said, "How will I ever learn how to get to where I need to go around here?"

Mrs. Breckinridge looked me straight in the eye and said, "Child, you've got a tongue, haven't you?"

I said, "Well, yes I do." I think that helped me probably more than anything else [she] ever did. I gave a simple answer but very much to the point. I never asked that question again!

Told by Gertrude Isaacs to Dale Deaton, November 15, 1978;
provided by the Louie B. Nunn Center for Oral History,
University of Kentucky Libraries, Lexington

Rats Making Noise

I always tell this story to my classes. It's not a Frontier Nursing Service story; it's a mountain story that illustrates so nicely my period of time and the differences between the inside and the outside. Moving ahead with the story, I took a lot of children to the oculist in Hazard, and one time I took a little preschooler from Confluence who was three or four years old. The nurse had identified something that was definitely wrong with her eyes.

Usually we didn't pick them up until they got to school, but this little girl was picked up because she couldn't read. Her family lived far back, and so I drove my jeep and picked up the mother, the nurse, the little girl, and another child. I took them to Dr. Cooley Comb's office in Hazard. He did all the examinations essentially free and then got us the glasses for these kids at cost. We did this through New Eyes for the Needy that gave us the money.

They put drops in this little girl's eyes while the nurse and her mother were sitting there with her, waiting for the drops to work and the doctor to come in. The doctor's receptionist was outside typing and the nurse, Cherry Evans, told me afterward that all of a sudden the little girl heard the typing and she turned to her mother and said, "Boy, them rats sure is chewing up that paper, ain't they?"

She had never seen a typewriter, so what she heard was the noise made by the lady typing on the paper!

Told by Dr. Mary Q. Hawkes, Newton, MA, to Dale Deaton,
June 16, 1979; provided by the Louie B. Nunn Center for
Oral History, University of Kentucky Libraries, Lexington

MOUNTAIN BOY'S FIRST TRIP TO A CITY

When I was taking a slew of kids to Cincinnati in a station wagon that was full of kids, and as I approached Cincinnati from the Kentucky side, I looked over and there was only one building I saw. I don't know whether it was the Carew Towers or the Sherry-Netherland [Hotel]. Anyhow, there was one building that was taller than the others, and about the only one of the skyline.

One little boy in the back seat looked over and sees this city, and being his first time out of the mountains, said, "Boy, you sure could hold a heap of hay in there."

What he said sure did tickle me.

Told by Dr. Mary Q. Hawkes, Newton, MA, to Dale Deaton,
June 16, 1979; provided by the Louie B. Nunn Center for
Oral History, University of Kentucky Libraries, Lexington

DOG HELPFUL AS A NURSE'S AIDE

I remember funny things that happened. Jean Holland was in the ward one day on the mothers' and babies' side. This is up in the old hospital, and Jean had this big golden retriever that wouldn't let Jean out of her sight. And this dog had snuck in because the living quarters were just through the door of the hospital. Well, the dog was under the bed in which Jean was giving this patient a bath, but Jean didn't know it.

All of a sudden the dog moved and she saw it. She said, "Missy, get out of here right now." Believe it or not, the patient's name was also Missy. Well, she tried to get out of the bed, but [couldn't]. . . .

Missy did a little bit of everything, and she was a good nurse's aide!

Told by Helen E. Browne, Wendover, to Dale Deaton, March 27, 1979;
provided by the Louie B. Nunn Center for Oral History,
University of Kentucky Libraries, Lexington

Rider Tossed from the Saddle

I was a volunteer courier at Frontier Nursing Services, although during that summer of 1964 I worked most of the time as a nurse's aide. One of my duties as a courier was to help exercise the horses. The nurses of FNS still did a few visits on horseback to some of the most remote areas of the county.

One day there was a little local boy that was going to help me by riding one horse while I rode the other. We left several horses in the barn; the horses we rode didn't like to leave the other horses. We were riding along and got started back. And just as soon as the horses in the barn heard us coming they started "whee-ing." Well, my horse took off in a gallop and my saddle slipped and I fell off. I wasn't hurt, but the little boy came up to me really frightened and said, "Are you kilt [killed] dead?"

I laughed and said, "I'm not kilt dead."

That summer at the Frontier Nursing Service was a good experience. It was fun and I learned a lot about the nursing care of mothers and babies. Along with my experiences at Hyden Hospital I also spent some time at Red Bird and Flat Creek, two of the six outpost centers.

Told by Martha Hill, Glendale, to Mark Brown, June 30, 2012;
provided by the Kentucky Historical Society, Frankfort

Nontalking Nurse Trainees

At Berea College we nursing students became very close. Although the class started with a larger number in 1962, there were only thirteen that graduated four years later. I don't know what happened to the ones that didn't graduate with us, but all of us in class were pretty close friends.

My roommate and I were not early morning people and we would get up, get dressed, and go to breakfast, then go to our work assignment at the hospital. We were never mad at each other but we just didn't talk a lot. I remember walking one day to our work assignment and we accidentally met up with another nursing student in our class. She was an early morning person and she talked, talked, talked, talked.

Finally both of us looked at her and said, "Would you please be quiet?"

I guess we weren't that awake yet and not ready to talk!

Told by Martha Hill, Glendale, to Mark Brown, June 30, 2012;
provided by the Kentucky Historical Society, Frankfort

Nurses Ate the Doctor's Cake

This is a memorable story about Dr. Robertson. It was his birthday, so we nurses put together our money to buy him a birthday cake. When he made the morning rounds we sang to him and presented his cake to him. I think he was pleased, even though he acted as if he didn't care. He took the cake back with him to his office to show his staff. Later that morning his office nurse brought the cake back to us, saying, "You all might as well go on and eat this cake because you know that Doc doesn't care a thing about things like this."

Well, about two-thirty in the afternoon we nurses cut the cake and began eating it. We thoroughly enjoyed each and every bite. In a short while we heard someone running up the steps, two at a time. It was Dr. Robertson's nurse, who said when she got to us, "Where is that cake? Doc wants to take it home to show his grandchildren."

We had just swallowed the last bite, which suddenly began growing larger and heavier in our stomachs. Wow, what an experience!

Evelyn Pearl Anderson, London, July 18, 2012

Lifelong Snuff Lover

The Centerville [Illinois] Township Hospital is the only place I ever worked that one could write on a time card, "Late because of train." I had to cross six railroad tracks to get from East Carondelet to Dupo on the main highway and then cross two more train tracks before getting to the hospital.

One evening while on duty in the ICU the nursing care staff was talking at the desk. The unit was designed in a circular fashion, with the most critical patients placed near the nurses' station desk. Immediately behind the desk was an elderly patient, a lady who was around eighty years old and was originally from Arkansas. She couldn't hear thunder; that is, until we talked softly at the desk! Then she heard every word and would enter into the discussion.

This lady loved snuff and would periodically call someone into her room to give her some snuff. When asked how long she had used snuff, she replied, "All of my life." Then she went on to say, "I used snuff when I was eight years old, and my daddy would take me out behind the house and whup me. I got married when I was thirteen, and my husband would catch me dipping snuff and he would take me out back and whup me."

I said, "You didn't learn a thing, did you?"
She responded with these words: "Nope, I sure like snuff."

Evelyn Pearl Anderson, London, July 18, 2012

WRONG PATIENT

This is a humorous story and I was so embarrassed when it happened. I hadn't been out of school very long and fact is, I may still have been in school. Numerous physicians back in those days were very intimidating. Well, back around 1961 one came up on the floor and he wanted to set up this lady for an exam, so she said, "Why does he want to do that?"

I said, "I really don't know but I guess he just wants to get everything checked out."

She said, "I'm having my tonsils taken out."

Well, he wanted a pelvic exam, and oh my gosh, no wonder she wondered! I had the wrong patient! [Heavy laughter.] I was so embarrassed.

Patricia A. Slater, Petersburg, March 6, 2013

THROWING DONUTS THROUGH WINDOWS

As a nurse I made my share of mistakes, such as when setting up your medications. You had to fill out an incident report if you made a mistake. However, I never did anything that was life threatening or was a major mistake. Most of the stories I know come from nurses that have to do things because you are nurses working in sometimes difficult situations. Some stories are just funny things that happen.

I worked several years in Labor and Delivery, often the night shift. One night one of the doctors came who had several women in labor [and] was spending the night in the doctor's lounge. About 2:00 a.m. he came out to the nurses' station and wanted to know if we were going to get some donuts. There was a bakery several miles from the hospital. The owner's wife had delivered at the hospital, and he would give us free donuts when we could pick them up. In those days you were not supposed to leave the hospital while on duty for any reason.

There were only two of us working that night, and we told him that we couldn't leave. Well, since all of the patients that night were his patients, he said, "Well, I'll watch the patients, so one of you go and get some donuts."

I had a car parked right outside the door into the unit. You had to go through the postpartum floor to get in and out. Going out was not a problem. When I returned the night supervisor was sitting at the desk on the postpartum unit. Well, I couldn't get in, as she would have known we had broken the rules. I went back out, and since my coworker was watching we decided that if we threw the donuts through the window, then I could come through as if I had been downstairs on a break.

It was summertime, so I just had to throw my purse and the bag of two dozen donuts through the window, which was about ten, twelve feet above the ground. The donuts were right in, so my coworker put them on the bed in the room. Next came my [purse], but the night supervisor was standing just outside the curtain in the room. The curtain was pulled back and the supervisor wanted to know, "What do you think you all are doing?"

My coworker's response was, "The doctor wanted some donuts." [Heavy laughter.] We were trying to shift the blame, that it was really his fault.

You should have seen us while we were laughing. I just couldn't get that purse through the window. I just kept hitting the wall!

Patricia A. Slater, Petersburg, March 6, 2013

THE THREE-H ASSIGNMENT

I was working Labor and Delivery at a time when many rural people still did not have indoor plumbing. One of the admitting procedures for these women was to get an enema so that the area remained clean during the delivery of the baby. One of the doctors that had a practice that served this population would joke, "Give them a three-H, it has been too cold to go to the outhouse." Three-H meant high, hot, and helluva lot!

Many years ago patients stayed in the hospital for weeks. Some actually lived in the hospital. The elderly, often with limited mobility, were constantly monitored by the head nurse and by the patients themselves, making sure their bowels were functioning with regularity. For some it is an obsession. We all have seen patients like this. On one unit the standard was on the third day, no BM [bowel movement], it was the 3H.

Patricia A. Slater, Petersburg, March 6, 2013

STUDENT'S SURPRISE BATH JOB

Student nurses at Berea College had to have their driver's license at the end of their junior year because they would be assigned a college vehicle to use to do public health nursing during their senior year. Mr. Kendall was our driver's education instructor. He economized by having one student drive while he was seated beside her. He would have two more students seated in the back as observers.

My friend Laurel was driving when she hit a pothole that sent our heads to the roof. It was a real waker-upper. Mr. Kendall exclaimed, "Miss Seals, be more careful! Pretend that you are driving a patient with appendicitis to the hospital and finish driving like that."

The next morning when I went on duty at the hospital, I was assigned to Mr. Kendall. He had been admitted overnight for an emergency appendectomy. The head nurse instructed that he was to have a complete bed bath. I was mortified to think that I had to give my instructor a complete bed bath. My face was flaming red with embarrassment when I took my pan of water to his bedside. Mr. Kendall said, "Miss Williams, just give me the washcloth and I will take care of things."

I was so relieved that I did not have to embarrass both of us by doing his private bath. However, his doctor ordered an enema. There was no getting out of that. I gave him the enema because I had to follow doctor's orders.

Mr. Kendall's son was not a nursing student but was my college classmate. Several years ago at a Berea College class reunion, I told him the above story. He started laughing and said, "Dad told me that story many times, but he didn't say who the student nurse was. Yeah, I have heard the same story from the other end!"

Clara Fay Smith, Erlanger, March 6, 2013

A MEMORABLE EVENT

I do remember what to me was a funny situation that took place in our clinical nursing checkoff. We had a list of procedures which we were to perform. When we had completed the procedure satisfactorily we were checked off on a printed list. "Checked off" meant the instructor would date and initial by the side of the written procedure. We could then perform the procedure without further observation or instruction. This included making beds, giving baths, or care, or anything or everything that required hands-on nursing care.

Our nursing arts instructor had been a military nurse. She was very methodical and exact in her training of us. The procedure which she was checking me off on was the proper way to administer a douche on a female patient. During the procedure, I had the nozzle inserted in such a way that the cleaning solution, which was basically water, accidentally sprayed up on the instructor's face. Oh, me, how terrible that was! When the procedure was completed and the patient was clean, dry, and comfortable in bed, I went to the utility room to clean the equipment. The instructor came to the door of the utility room and said to me, "Miss Carpenter, that patient had syphilis."

I said, "Yes, ma'am, I know."

You would have had to have known the instructor to know how funny this seemed at the time. Of course, I didn't laugh at the time. There was not a bad outcome. It was just unfortunate and memorable.

Evelyn Pearl Anderson, London; reprinted from Anderson,
Daylite's A-Comin' *(Baltimore: Publish America, 2007), 38*

DIRECTIONS MISINTERPRETED

If you could find them, there are interesting stories coming from home health or hospice, without revealing names. These might include how directions to homes are written by one and interpreted by another, such as, "Go to the black church and turn right," leaving the nurse who had moved in from the northern part of the United States to drive around a village for two hours before calling in to the office to say she couldn't find a single church that was painted black.

Truth of the matter is that it was an African American church, typically known as a "black church."

Evelyn Pearl Anderson, London, March 27, 2013

ODD NAME FOR A TRUCK

A trucker was driving through Bowling Green and was hospitalized because he had injured his back when he stepped down out of the truck. He was my patient for several days and we talked about a lot of things about his family, life, etc. I felt sorry for him because he was going to be in the hospital for several days, so I took his clothes home and washed them.

One day he asked me if I would tell him my first name. I told him my name was Jenny and he said, "You're kidding, that's my truck's name!"

Jenny Burton, Bowling Green, May 8, 2013

Request for a Watch

One of my many nursing positions through the 1980s was the role of patient education for a medium-size hospital. Cardiac teaching was one of several offered modules and was physician-ordered for patients after a heart attack.

One patient I remember quite well. Entering her senior years and hailing from a rural area not too far away. My goal for teaching her the next day would be for her to learn to take her pulse. As I left her room I asked her to have one of her family members to bring her a wristwatch with a second hand for the next day's lesson. The following day, when entering her room, I asked if the family had found a watch for her to use. Immediately I saw a confused expression on her face.

She said they called to say that all their watches had two hands. Needless to say, I loaned her mine.

Theresa Sue Milburn King, Danville, June 18, 2013

Oops, Nurse's Mistake

The small hospital where I first worked handled everything from birth to death and most surgeries and traumas in between. Usually only one registered nurse worked each shift and was expected to be in charge of it all, including all hospitalized patients as well as those in labor and delivery and in the emergency room.

One busy three-to-eleven shift found me with one lady in labor and her doctor present but in surgery. I diligently held the woman's hand and gave her words of encouragement. Not fully yet understanding the precision of vaginal exams to check for the progress of labor, I still kept the doctor apprised of progress while he was operating.

The contractions, of course, became closer and closer, and the doctor was still operating when she screamed, "The baby is coming!" So I decided to take another look, and sure enough, she was crowning. I ran to the surgery suite, yelling, "I see the head! I see the head!"

Thankfully the doctor was finishing his case and soon appeared in the labor room. As instructed, my patient was taken to the delivery room. As the baby was coming into the world, the doctor looked over at frantic me and asked, "Did they teach you anatomy at your university?"

Of course, I said, "Yes."

He responded, "Well, this is not the baby's head, but the little boy's scrotum!"

There's no fool like a young fool, and I heard about my "mix-up" for days.

Theresa Sue Milburn King, Danville, June 18, 2013

A PROFESSIONAL ERROR

For more than fourteen years I have worked in a clinic here in Kentucky. When I started I was only twenty-one years of age. To this day, this clinic still generates off paper charting. So when a patient comes in the nurse fills out what we call an encounter form. At the top of the form is the patient's name, date of birth, date, medication, and reason for the visit.

I had just started working in the back, triaging patients for a certain doctor. I assume my nerves were wearing on me that day I checked in a middle-age guy. On the encounter form we have to write the patient's name, first and last. So I checked the gentleman in and his complaint was gout. I finished triaging him and then went on to check the next patient. I was so happy with my job because I was finally doing what I had been wanting to do for a long time—patient care. I heard my name being called from the doctor's office. I went to his office and the doctor I was working for was laughing. He said, "Come here and look at this." It was the encounter form I had just filled out on the gentleman with gout.

I looked at what the doctor was pointing at. I had written down "gout" for the patient's last name!

Needless to say, we had to change it. We still joke about it until this day!!

Dana Burnam, Bowling Green, July 28, 2013

NORMAL VERSUS ABNORMAL

One day I called a patient about his lab results. The gentleman answered the phone and I asked for him. He replied, "This is he."

After telling him his test results were all normal, he then asked, "What's normal?" Without thinking about it, I replied, "Well, if your tests weren't normal, then they would be abnormal."

I don't know what I was thinking that day, because after I said it I was so embarrassed. I kept saying to myself, that didn't make sense at all, or maybe the patient thought I didn't know what I was talking about.

Dana Burnam, Bowling Green, July 29, 2013

STRANGE VERBAL REQUESTS

At the Gowan Nursing Home in Robinson, Illinois, one of the elderly men kept yelling repeatedly, "Oh dear, my back! Oh dear, my back!" I went down to his room and gave him a back rub to try to calm him. Later I heard again, "Oh dear, my back!" So I went and talked to him for a while and he finally asked me my name.

Next time, he began to yell, "Oh dear, Charlene!"

Another little lady would repeat, "Hurry up, cuppy kay; hurry up, cuppy kay," to no one in particular. I wondered if she was meaning cupcake but was told that was not the case. It was something she had invented.

Charlene Vaught, Portland, TN, August 2, 2011

5

PATIENT MISBEHAVIOR

Typically, misbehavior by patients, nurses, or doctors is not spoken or written about. However, inappropriate situations do occur, whether through thoughts, smiles, stubbornness, noises, or various life-threatening events. Some of the events these stories recount involve relatively minor tomfoolery or refusal to comply with medical advice, while others touch on more serious ethical breaches. Some even illustrate a more profound clash of values, as in one nurse's sympathetic account of a patient who strenuously resisted the efforts of nuns to "convert" her before death.

IMPROPER LOCATION OF FALSE TEETH

After finishing nurses training I found a job at Pleasant Acres Nursing Home in Altamont, Illinois. During my orientation as a new nurse I had to have a week not only following the other nurses on their routines but also the activity director, whose early morning duties included shaving the men.

I had never shaved a man before but figured it couldn't be too difficult an undertaking. Was I ever wrong! I proceeded to shave this old gentleman who apparently had not yet put his false teeth in place. Besides that, he kept moving his mouth in a chewing motion the entire time I was trying to shave him.

Needless to say, that little incident tired me out for the whole shift.

Charlene Vaught, Portland, TN, August 2, 2011

THE WOMAN WHO WOULDN'T

As I entered the room the patient in bed 303 looked directly at me with a smugly satisfied smile. Her smile was not the usual facial expression one sees in a hospitalized woman who has advanced cirrhosis of the liver.

Puzzled, I continued and introduced myself as the in-charge nurse for the afternoon. As I spoke I noticed her bloated face, pasty white pallor, and abdomen too large for her thin legs and arms. Purple striate mottled the glistening taut skin, and her umbilicus [belly button] had disappeared with the distention. Liver failure, I mentally recorded. Her appearance fit the nursing shift report of a patient in rapid physical decline, but her demeanor seemed disconnected from this reality. Being trained to search until the pieces fit my nursing instinct on alert, I knew my assessment was incomplete.

She spoke up and said to me, "I hope you are not here to convert me! I have had enough of that tactic."

I said, "What do you mean, convert you?"

She said, "Haven't you heard my story yet? The good nuns want me to reject my twenty-year marriage, then ask the priest for absolution and sprinkle holy water on me while I beg for salvation."

"Why would they want you to do that?" I asked her.

"Because I live in a second marriage and it is unholy in the eyes of the good nuns," she disgustedly grimaced. "It's like this. I was a practicing Catholic when I married my first husband, and we had a miserable marriage so we divorced. Nevertheless, in the eyes of the Catholic Church I now live in adultery. So the nuns come daily to my room, pray over me, and beg my repentance. But I will have none of it." Her bellowing voice left no doubt of the pending outcome.

When she spoke, her short, thinning brown hair seemed to become alert. In a nebulous way she appeared jovial about the rebellious encounter. Her mannerisms conveyed that she was enjoying the attention and the opportunity to declare her right to self-determination. As her body failed daily, without reprieve, I wondered if this power struggle represented one last opportunity to gain control over her fate. I said to her, "That must be uncomfortable."

Her response was, "You better believe it! But that's enough for today. I think I need a nap."

"I will be back to check on you, but let me know if you need something sooner, or if you want to talk."

Mrs. Thompson, which was her name, lay on the bed and slept soundly.

In sharp contrast, the nuns were distraught. Each afternoon on the six following days they came to the unit to ask about Mrs. Thompson's health, and when Mrs. Thompson allowed it they met with her. When they stepped off the hospital elevator their sorrowful countenance cast a heaviness that permeated the ward. Our bodies felt heavier. The nuns walked slowly, with hands folded, heads bent forward, seemingly deep in contemplation, praying for guidance, certain that it was their heavy burden to ensure this woman did not die unrepented and find herself burning in hell forever. It was their duty to find the right words, to pray the right prayer in order to achieve the right miracle even at the last minute before her physical survival slipped away. And so it went, until one afternoon during the next week I learned in the shift report that Mrs. Thompson had gone to her residential home. Silently I prayed for her well-being.

My next encounter with Mrs. Thompson was one month later. As night supervisor for the midnight shift my routine first action duty was to personally visit every room of the three-floor hospital. In the past there had been several incidents when I or another nurse went into a room only to find someone in trouble. Twice in the last year we found patients sitting in a chair, dead. Things could happen after I visited the rooms, but at least I knew what was happening at the start of the shift.

Halfway through the visitations, my pager sounded an alarm code that I knew meant for me to come quickly. I followed the code direction to the floor above, headed for Mrs. Thompson's room. When I got there the excited nurse said, "Mrs. Thompson fell from the bed," as she pointed to a room two doors away. [The] image I saw when I stepped into the room is seared forever into my mind. On the floor, a hospital gown only half-covering the intended areas, suspended by the still-connected IV tubing to both bed and her left arm, sat Mrs. Thompson with hair disheveled, wide-eyed, weak but defiant. Her eyes had lost the previous luster but the fight was still there. Her whole demeanor spoke the message, "I may die and I may die soon, but I will die without yielding to the will of others. Damn the world, damn the fact that alcohol caused my illness, damn the fact that I married outside of the church! Damn this bed that won't keep me from the floor. I am who I am and shall continue my sense of self."

She calmed as we returned her to bed, repositioned all the hospital gadgets, pulled the sidebars up, and once again made her bed a safe haven. Her eyes met mine and remained fixed. She said to me, "They've won, you know."

I replied, "I know that is very important to you. How can I help you?"

She firmed her grip on my hand and said, "Just be you."

When she said that, a tear fell from my eye. There was no stopping it. I reached down and gave her a hug and said, "You hang on to that bed the rest of the night. Okay?"

Mrs. Thompson raised her unbridled hand, thumb up, signaled victory, and replied, "You bet!"

Her condition progressively worsened during the following days. That handshake she always offered gradually weakened, and as the weakness progressed her flaccid body seemed to absorb the mattress upon which she lay. The liver, drowned by alcohol, continued to lose its life-giving cells, and her near destiny was now obvious to all.

The nuns pleaded, "With only a few hours or days left to live, what will it hurt to say you are not going to live as a married woman any longer? Just do this and you can be buried in hallow dirt blessed with holy water, by a holy priest. Do this and you shall see God and live in perfect bliss for eternity. Surely admitting the need to abide by the rules of the Catholic Church is worth this." A blast of hot air visibly burst across the room as a clear, relentless, and definite NO rang out.

She wouldn't and she didn't, so she died without repent. She was buried in an unholy mound of dirt without blessing from the Catholic Church. She left the nuns with a sense of failure. So where now does the spirit of the "Woman Who Wouldn't" live? In some way it lives in all [persons] who shared her life experience. I am confident she died firmly believing that she had stayed true to herself despite the prayers and coercion. One could not help but respect her emotional strength. I also wondered if standing so firm was worth the price. Perhaps the nuns' healing rituals would have brought comfort, even in the face of nonbelief. It later struck me that I had never met her husband. I was left wondering if her prize of self-control was ultimately a win.

As so many times before, to stay in nursing I had to make sense of the spiritual dilemma. Wrestling with my personal questioning, I sought internal peace. To quiet this need for answers my final resolution was simply to name the paradox. Mrs. Thompson's strong sense of self-direction gathered the courage she needed to fight the Catholic Church even as she died and gave her dignity as she lost her life. She won her battle with the good nuns. Her strong sense of self-direction in the face of evidence [about the dangers] also led her to embrace alcohol and killed her.

Who won? I can't answer this existential question. Perhaps we all won. Perhaps the struggle was merely a life play, with each person acting their prescribed life role. Perhaps in what seemed . . . defeat the nuns claimed self-respect, as they gave their best efforts to save Mrs. Thompson's eternal soul.

What I know with certainty was that as a nurse I was required to honor the preciousness of Mrs. Thompson's life, no matter how she chose to live it. To the best of my ability I played my role.

Dr. Kay T. Roberts, Louisville, December 17, 2011;
initially published by Women Who Write in Calliope, 2011;
publication permission not needed, but granted

YOUNG PATIENT'S MISBEHAVIOR

I was working from 11:00 p.m. to 7:00 a.m. in the pediatric intensive care unit at UK medical center, and on one occasion I bent over to pick up something beside a child's bed when I was pinched on the fanny. I looked around, even though I knew that no one else was there except three sleeping children. It happened again soon afterward.

I realized it was one of the children, who was small for his age and a patient in the ICU.

Jo Ann M. Wever, Springfield, March 14, 2012

HALCION EVENT

One long night shift, another nurse and I had eighteen patients each, not uncommon in those days, unlike today, where the nurse-patient ratios actually exist. We had made our first rounds, and since it was about 2:00 a.m. we started hearing strange sounds coming from one of the hallways. Keep in mind that this floor was called bedpan alley by the nurses, since the youngest patient was sixty years old—not so old to a lot of us anymore! The other nurse—let's call her Mary, a nice, general name, like Jane, so as to not offend anyone—and I started down the hall to pinpoint the sounds. Remember, back then everyone received back rubs and Halcion at 9:00 p.m., and by 11:00 p.m. all were ready for sleep except the sundowners. The noise would start and stop, so it was hard to pin down. Just when we thought we had the banging rails, yelling, cursing, and the scraping of furniture [pinned] down to which room it was coming from, it would stop. We looked in all the rooms around close to the area we thought the sound was from and finally found one in which I thought the entire bed had been removed. By this time everything was getting funny and the sound was still going on at 4:00 a.m., when all strange things go on in a hospital.

A plan was made for the capture of the villain for the sounds which went creak in the night. Patient rounds were quickly made and then we set up on each side of the door to catch the action as it occurred. It did occur, with loud banging, squeaking, cursing, and yelling begun. We threw the door open and found a naked man "fighting the Germans" with his IV pole, fluids swinging wildly from side to side, tubing pulled tight, with the bed in the middle of the room, using the trapeze bar and the traction frame, we assumed, as the side of his "foxhole." He was cursing and showing us everything he had, and to me, as a newer nurse, I was welcomed into the real world of nursing quite quickly.

After this encounter with Halcion, Ativan became my best friend to suggest to residents and physicians alike.

Jana Buckles, Lawrenceburg, June 6, 2012

A Stubborn Woman

This is about a noncompliant lady that I inherited soon after I arrived on a certain district. I had only maybe met her one time when she called in labor, and we really didn't know each other. So she didn't have any confidence in me because I wasn't the nurse she had been seeing. I don't know how she was with that nurse and I never did find out, but wish I had. When I went to her house [and she was] in labor, she was totally uncooperative in breathing or anything, and she finally got out of control and was screaming and jumping around in the bed. Well, that lengthens your labor, not shorten[s] it. One needs to buckle down in laboring; that means working, but she wasn't doing it, and even her husband yelled at her from the other room, "Shut up and do what she told you." But she didn't do it.

Anyway, the baby was eventually delivered but I don't know who was more exhausted, her or me. The baby was fine, so we did our thing, and it was not the most healthy household, but I went away and tried to get some shut-eye and then went back early the next morning, but there was no place for me to park the jeep right there. I had to park it elsewhere and walk a little bit, but for some reason there wasn't a dog there, which is unusual. The next result was that I was on her front porch before she knew I was there, and I heard this movement of feet across the floor, so I yelled and when she said, "Come in," I opened the door and went in. The mop bucket was sitting in the middle of the floor with the mop in it. The floor was sopping wet, the mother is in bed, and the bed is still bouncing. So I pulled back the covers and saw her soaking-wet feet. She had been up mopping the floor.

So I delivered my best lecture on that. Bear in mind that out of the mountains you kept people in bed for a week after childbirth at that time. We now know better, but I don't think anybody recommends mopping with a bucket. The very next morning I said to her, "You don't have to be doing that. Let it stay dirty if you haven't got somebody that'll come and do it for you. It wasn't that dirty anyway."

So she checked out all right and I went about my business. The next morning I went back at a slightly different hour and there was no mop bucket in sight but the floor was wet and her feet were wet. I said, "Okay, now, six weeks from today you will be at my door saying, 'Nurse, how come my back hurts all the time?' You are going to have to quit this."

Six weeks to the day she's back at the clinic and asked, "Nurse, how come my back hurts all the time?"

She was a noncompliant patient. She looked after her baby very well, which was the big thing, but she didn't look after herself. She was making sure her house floor was clean, and to her that was more important than her health. I have a problem with that priority, but apparently she didn't.

Told by Jean Fee to Rebecca Adkins Fletcher, June 15, 2002;
provided by the Louie B. Nunn Center for Oral History,
University of Kentucky Libraries, Lexington

YOUNG MAN THREATENS NURSES

There were people I worked with that had some significant impressions, even threats. I think this happened to me and my nurse friend Betty Lester, but it might not have been her. Anyway, we got a call one night and went way up a creek to get to where [we] were scheduled.

There was a young man of seventeen with his wife in eclampsia, pregnant. And he stood there with a shotgun, facing us, and said, "If she dies, you die." We remained there about twenty-four hours before we got released.

So that was truly an interesting experience.

Told by Anne Winslow to Anne Campbell Ritchie, September 25, 1979;
provided by the Louie B. Nunn Center for Oral History,
University of Kentucky Libraries, Lexington

BAD AND GOOD BEHAVIOR

There was one patient that I had one time while I was still a nurse student. I was trying to get him up and get him to walk a little and then he started hitting me with his cane. And I said, "Don't you do that."

Well, he didn't, but I thought I was going to get socked over my arm or back with his cane, but it didn't go that far.

After I graduated and was working at Methodist Hospital I worked with a difficult patient and none of the nurses there enjoyed taking care of this fellow. He was sort of obnoxious and would cuss at you when you went in to help him. He would be on his call light all the time wanting this or that. The other patients in the room did not like his behavior either.

One day a lightbulb sort of lit up in my head and I thought about a film we had seen in nursing school called *Mrs. Reynolds Needs a Nurse*. Basically, that film showed that she was really afraid of dying while being alone. So I thought to myself about this man and wondered if his problem was the same as Mrs. Reynolds's. He was afraid of dying.

I went in and talked with him but don't remember what all I said, but it became sort of a personal challenge, so I started taking care of him when I was working and [would] go in often to do things for him. After that he became a very good patient for me and I remember when he did die I cried along with his family. I truly missed him because I had gotten so close to him after realizing that was the cause of his anxiety; he was afraid of dying.

I hope I helped him have a peaceful death with the care I gave him.

Told by Martha Hill, Glendale, to Mark Brown, June 30, 2012;
provided by the Kentucky Historical Society, Frankfort

DELIRIOUS PATIENT

There was a man who had been admitted to the hospital with multiple fractures of his ribs, hip, and leg resulting from a tractor accident. He was in the bed, harnessed in traction equipment. One morning he attempted to get out of bed on his own. In fact, he was on his way over the protective bed railing.

He was totally out of his head, as much as his head was out of the bed. Upon questioning his wife I learned that the man consumed alcohol regularly and compulsively. The wife failed to relay this information on his admission, . . . thinking it was not important. The man was having delirium tremens from abstinence [from] alcohol.

Needless to say, it was an interesting few hours with his yelling and fighting against us.

The physician successfully sedated the patient. I think this was my first experience in observing delirium tremens. It seemed to be an appropriate name for what I observed—a patient in tremors deliriously.

Evelyn Pearl Anderson, London, July 18, 2012

ALCOHOLIC PATIENT

One particular night we had admitted an alcoholic and had orders to watch for tremors and DTs [delirium tremens]. I came to work the next day and walked into his room. He was sitting up in his bed next to the headboard. He was taking his pillow and hitting the bed with it, so I asked him what was wrong.

He said, "Are you blind? Look at them huge spiders. Don't you see them, since they are all over the bed and climbing on the walls?" I ran out of the room and called his doc, who ordered Valium and a shot of whiskey. When I went back to the room to take care of him he had barricaded all the doors and had lost everything by throwing furniture around the room.

We called the cops to help us get in the room, and they had to remove the door from the hinges in order to get to him. Needless to say, they took him out in handcuffs because they were afraid he was going to hurt the nurses.

Teresa Fryman Bell, Edmonson County, October 29, 2012

EARLY NURSE EXPERIENCE

My first nursing job after I received my BS in nursing degree from Berea College was at Booth Memorial Hospital in Covington, Kentucky. My husband's parents lived in eastern Kentucky, in Estill County. When my mother-in-law was diagnosed with breast cancer, my father-in-law asked me to choose the surgeon. I recommended Dr. Vesper, who was one of the surgeons with whom I worked.

After her surgery she was put in a room on the unit where I was assistant head nurse. Much to my dismay, my mother-in-law was a heavy smoker. In those days smokers were allowed to smoke in their rooms.

Several days post op, I had assigned a student nurse to take care of Mom.

In the middle of a busy morning someone came running to tell me that there was a fire in her room. I called the fire department and we quickly extinguished the fire before the fire department arrived. However, the fire department came and investigated as a precaution. I was so embarrassed that Mom's smoking was the cause of the fire.

She knew how upset I was with her and she tried to defend herself by saying, "It wasn't my fault. The student nurse emptied my ashtray into the garbage can."

I responded by saying, "If you hadn't been smoking it would not have happened at all." To say the least, this was a bit of a touchy family situation.

Clara Fay Smith, Erlanger, March 6, 2013

Training on the Psychiatric Unit

Psychiatry was really a new experience for me. I knew nothing about it but was about to learn. We had classes both in and out of our work areas. It was interesting but not my favorite place to be. The hospital was divided into acute, chronic, and convalescent units for male [patients], and the same for female. The six units are what I remember. I liked the acute male unit the best and disliked the convalescent female unit.

On one of our introductory tours as part of our orientation, an instructor took us to the chronic female unit. When she opened the door about ten of us entered. A little nun patient seated alongside of the left wall exclaimed, "Hello, hello, World War III, they're coming, they're coming, about three thousand of them."

Well, we didn't know what to think! We continued our tour somewhat shaken but never to forget that moment. I recall that I received good reviews on all the floors [units] I worked.

My first assignment was the psychiatric acute male unit. I do not recall having a patient who became unmanageable. I administered their medication and talked with them as they played cards. I knew that you had to be on guard. There were true stories about a man who quietly entered the nurses' station and dropped scales on the nurse's head while she was charting, so I knew to be cautious.

One Sunday afternoon I had a patient escape through the entrance door. He slipped out as an employee unlocked the door and entered. I saw him leave, so off I went after him. I ran past the orderly, telling him to watch the others. I ran past the switchboard operator, located off the lobby, asking him to send some help. Out the front door and into the bright sunshine I went with my snow-white uniform, white stockings, and sparkling-white Clinic brand lace-up shoes with snow-white shoestrings and my white cap on. Quite a dazzling sight, I am sure.

Our Lady of Peace was on a hill. Well, to get to [the] runaway patient, I had to run down the hill to Newburg Road. The patient was standing on the side of the road but he did not try to harm me. He did not try to run from me. I looked back toward the hospital to see if any help was coming. What I saw surprised me. It was an orderly running down the hill to help, which was no surprise. The surprise was that every window in [the] front of the hospital had at least two or three heads in it. Thus we had quite an audience.

The patient picked up rocks alongside of the road and began throwing them at the orderly. He never threw one at me. I walked toward the patient very slowly, as did the orderly. We were able to get him back up the hill to the hospital without problems.

Once back on the unit, the patient quietly went to his room. At the evening meal, the patient was overheard saying to another patient, "Bill, if I had my car out back like you are going to have when you leave here tomorrow, that little nurse would have never caught me!"

Evelyn Pearl Anderson, London; reprinted from Anderson,
Daylite's A-Comin' *(Baltimore: Publish America, 2007), 62–63*

IMPROPER WORDS

An older gentleman who was unable to retain urine had to wear a Texas catheter, which is a condom-type catheter that is placed over the penis, and it has a tube [that] goes to the bedside to collect the urine.

He continued to remove it, and while [I was] trying to replace it he would fight me and yell, "You are nothing but an ol' whore, so leave my pecker alone!"

Jenny Burton, Bowling Green, May 8, 2013

ALCOHOL PROBLEM

A man was admitted for back pain and placed in pelvic traction for treatment. He had a history of drinking a six-pack daily, and part of the doctor's orders was that he could have three beers a day when requesting it.

One evening when [I was] making rounds he was out of traction, and when asked what he was doing he stated he was going. When I asked him where he was going, he immediately charged at me like a bull and pinned me up against the door frame. There was a visitor in the hall, so I yelled for him to get me some help.

[It] took seven or eight people to wrestle that man down and give him sedation. We called his brother to tell him his brother had gone into DTs. When he came to see him he was afraid I was going to have him arrested, so I said I should but would not, then went on to say, "But he needs help with his alcohol problem."

Jenny Burton, Bowling Green, May 8, 2013

STUDENT'S PSYCHIATRIC PATIENT

I went to Eastern State Psychiatric Hospital in Lexington for some of my psychiatric clinical experiences. While I was there in the clinical area I had a patient whose diagnosis, I think, was catatonic. While in psych we always used our last name and that was how our name tags were printed, and we were not to give patients any personal information about ourselves. Our clinical objective was to get them to talk and tell us what bothered them.

After the experience was over I got a card and letter from my patient. He had addressed it to Miss Ulm, Berea College, Berea, KY. That really frightened me because I thought that he knew my name and where I was going to school, so he might come looking for me.

Well, thank goodness he never did, but that was another reason that made me dislike psychiatric nursing.

Told by Martha Hill, Glendale, to Mark Brown, June 30, 2012;
provided by the Kentucky Historical Society, Frankfort

6

Inspirational Tales

The nurse-patient relationship can be inspirational for either party. In this chapter, many nurses describe patient's inspirational words or actions. A truly inspirational story describes the nurse who frequently held hands with dying patients. In nursing homes, when newcomers enter, all staff members know they need to interact with them to make them feel comfortable, almost as if they were in a new home. To do so helps the new patients continue being as active as possible on a daily basis.

Numerous stories in this chapter talk about Mary Breckinridge, founder of the Frontier Nursing Service, especially how she inspired various nurses, midwives, and Appalachian Mountain residents to become reliable, dedicated servants for those in need of food, clothing, shelter, and so on. Other stories speak of church pastors and missionaries, as well as loving services in honor of the Lord.

A Life's Lesson

I met a man who was a patient in the hospital where I began my nursing career. He was one of those sweet little elderly persons with eyes that sparkled. He always grinned from ear to ear. On one occasion I was assigned to be his student nurse. For privacy reasons, I will refer to him as Mr. P. I truly enjoyed taking care of Mr. P. To this day, after twenty-two years of hospital nursing, I still remember him, and when I think of him I smile.

After I graduated from nursing school I became an employee at that same hospital. One day when I cared for Mr. P. he wanted a shave. Well, I was still quite a young, new nurse, just starting out, you might say, and I wasn't too sure about the shaving procedure. We just didn't do that much shaving in nursing school. We learned all the other hygiene pretty well—bedpans, bed making, bed baths, etc.

I thought that I would try to shave him, but how do I go about this? The best thing I did was to be honest with Mr. P. and tell him I wasn't too sure how to do it. Without any hesitation he said, "I'll just talk you through it." All of this time he was still smiling with a big, loving smile. (I sit here smiling too as I think back to that time many years ago.)

So Mr. P. got his shave and I received a checkoff on a new procedure. We both did just fine, and then he reminded me of another lesson in life as I commented on his smile. He grinned really big and said, "Well, I think if you just keep smiling, the whole world will smile back."

Rebecca Collins, Auburn, September 14, 2011

"I Feel Pretty, Too"

As a retired registered nurse I have turned my patient-care skills into gardening skills for my one acre [of] land. Recently while working in the yard I was reminded of a wonderful lady whom I had only known for a year. She used to love to keep a garden and would always home can the fruits of her labors. I firmly believe God has a purpose for each and every one of us. It may not be the purpose for which we asked, but it is the purpose he wants us to have. I also firmly believe every person we meet in life makes an impact on the outcome of our lives. People we have known for only a short time can make a lasting impression on the way we want our lives to be. Gladys Alexander, known as Mrs. A. to her caregivers, was one of those rare persons who drift into your life, steal your heart, then drift out again.

After September 11, 2011, my nursing career shifted from delivering babies to taking care of the elderly. I really needed a change, so after fifteen years of working night shift I finally had the opportunity to work day shift in my hometown hospital. Naturally, I was not sure if I could switch from newborn babies to adults, because some habits are hard to break. After six months I learned I did not like taking care of medical-surgical patients, but I did not want to give up my day job.

God answered my prayers when he sent me a challenge. I accepted an administration job in the extended care facility of the same hospital. I had always said I would never work in a nursing home, but I should have known to never say "never." Just two days on the job, one resident had already wormed her way into my heart. By the time I met Mrs. A. she was totally dependent on her caregivers for all her needs, but just because she was incapacitated did not mean she was less of a person.

Mrs. A. loved to talk about her children and grandchildren, and she loved to talk about gardening and canning.

Almost every day Mrs. A. could be found sitting in the hall watching all the daily activities and people going by. I loved to stop and talk with her and one day I commented on how pretty she looked. She replied to my comments by saying, ". . . and I feel pretty, too."

From that day on I never failed to tell Mrs. A. how pretty she was and she never failed to say, "I feel pretty, too." Her simple statement said so much about her character. Here was a woman who had been bed-bound for many years but her sense of self-worth was still intact.

We lost Mrs. A. in 2003 but she will live on as a strong woman with a flourishing self-esteem and an overwhelming feeling of love for her family. So the next time someone pays you a compliment, just smile at them and say, ". . . and I feel pretty, too."

Goodbye, Mrs. A., you are truly missed.

Bobbi Dawn Rightmyer, Harrodsburg, February 22, 2012

DO BAD THINGS REALLY HAPPEN IN THREES?

I have never really considered myself a superstitious person, even though I do have a few little idiosyncrasies, but there are many people who do believe in all types of superstitions. My Granny Sallee tried to never enter through a door she had not exited from because that was considered to be bad luck. My Granny Devine hated for a black cat to cross her path, as that was also considered bad luck. And what child has not secretly "stepped on a crack" when they were upset with their mother? However, there is one superstition-like occurrence I do believe in, and that is, bad things come in threes.

Have you ever noticed how everything bad in your life always seems to happen in threes? As a nurse I could probably ramble off all kinds of instances of bad things happening in my life in threes. But the "bad" threes I want to tell about have actually been blessings that passed ever so briefly through my life while working in the local extended care unit of the local hospital. Even though I only knew these persons for a short while, all three left a lasting impression on my life.

Jesse was number one, as he was such a wonderful man. He never complained and always had a quick smile. The Kentucky Wildcats were his favorite pastime, next to visiting with his family. Jesse's family visited every day and not a single day went by when someone didn't come to see him. His family was dedicated, and they taught me just how loyal your family can be.

When Jesse died it was sudden but not unexpected, and I think the entire staff mourned in silence as we tried to carry on with work as usual, except it was not work as usual. I do not think there is a nurse out there who does not believe that deaths happen in threes, especially in a hospital. The staff was suddenly looking for any unusual aches, pains, or other symptoms of impending illness in all the patients. Who would be the next to go?

Number two happened exactly one week later. Nancy Katherine was secretly one of my favorites and I would have probably done anything in the world for her. You know how you sometimes take an instant liking to someone and all you want to do is help him or her out. That was how I felt about Nancy Katherine. She was so set in her ways that everything in her life had to be just like it was the day before and the day before that and the day before that. I know I am going to be just like her when I get older! She did not like things to change and neither do I.

Nancy Katherine never called me by my name, thus to her I was always "Dr. Rightmyer's daughter." My father-in-law had been the favorite local dentist and this is how she chose to remember me. Every day she always had a hug for me, and now I'm going to miss our special time together. The problem was, I didn't have near enough time to grieve for her because number three happened three days later.

Frank was such a quiet man, but he will be greatly missed. He never complained about anything or anyone because he was just happy about everything you did for him. He always went to church on Sundays, and up until the end he participated in all types of activities. Anyone could say, "How are you doing, Frank?" And he always answered, "I'm all right."

It was strange for a while with those three not around. There was no Jesse to tell you the score of the game, no Nancy to say, "Will you be my nurse?," and no Frank to make you appreciate the imperfections of life. It was hard for a short time to see someone else living in those three rooms, but eventually other people entered our lives. The new people needed us as much as the three did, and they also wormed their way right into my heart.

Do bad things really happen in threes? I still believe that, but in this case my three "bads" turned out to be blessings in disguise. I was able to give these three a small amount of comfort during their remaining days and they were able to give me a better appreciation of life. And you know what else, I think there are three new angels in heaven looking down on all of us with smiles on their faces and happiness in their hearts. Goodbye, my angels, you will truly be missed.

Bobbi Dawn Rightmyer, Harrodsburg, February 28, 2012

GARDENING WITH SPECIAL NEEDS

It takes a special kind of person to be a nurse in a nursing home or assisted living facility. The patients in these institutions have been moved from their homes and are now living a life that is much different from what they were accustomed to. Many families feel forced to move loved ones into these facilities when the burden of care at home becomes too much. Then it is up to the nurses to provide a loving, safe, and fulfilling home for these people.

The last five years of my nursing career were spent working on a thirty-five-bed extended care facility located in the upstairs of my local hospital. We always ran at full capacity, thus there were thirty-five individual patients we had to try and care for. One of my jobs as the assessment coordinator was to work with the social worker and activity director to provide a home-like environment for these patients.

Upon initial assessment with the patient and their family it was my job to find out what their daily routine was while they were living at home. Were they early risers or late sleepers? What was their biggest meal of the day? What activities did they look forward to every day? These are just a few of the important questions we would try to piece together in order to plan the appropriate care for the patient.

During my second spring working in extended care I had several patients who missed working in their gardens at home, so we decided to plant gardens at the hospital. After obtaining the proper permission we arranged to have four iron tables bought for a corner of the back parking lot and placed a hard-shelled children's swimming pool on each table. We filled the pools with soil and bought the plants . . . which our patients had requested.

On a warm spring morning we brought six of our patients down to the new garden in their wheelchairs. Having the pools up on the tables made it easy for the patients to reach the dirt and help plant the vegetables. We planted tomatoes, onions, lettuce, cucumbers, and beans, along with a few marigolds to help keep the bugs away. Someone had donated two half-whiskey barrels, and we planted these with tobacco transplants because we had a patient who missed working in his tobacco.

All summer long patients would take turns during the day to go downstairs to help in the garden. It was my duty every morning before coming upstairs to make sure the plants were watered, then after breakfast the ladies and one gentleman would come outside and tend to the garden, picking the ripe vegetables and snipping off dead leaves and blooms.

The dietician at the hospital was really good about working with the patients and using their vegetables for meals or for snack time. If we were lucky enough to have lots of tomatoes one day the patients may have bacon, lettuce, and tomato sandwiches for lunch. Many times a mess of greens would be served up with supper. The ladies enjoyed "snapping" beans and would line up in the hallways of the facility with their bean bowls and scrap buckets.

The gentleman with the tobacco was thrilled to see his tobacco grow, and he loved working the fertilizer into the soil. Because of his limited ability to stand without assistance he trusted me to "top" his tobacco under his close supervision. In the fall when the tobacco was ready to be cut, the gentleman's nephew brought in an old tobacco knife and we cut down the ten stalks of tobacco. We didn't have any tobacco sticks, but we did use wire coat hangers to hang the tobacco in an old storage closet until it was ready to be stripped. At stripping time this gentleman sat in his chair all day and carefully stripped the leaves, graded the tobacco, and hand-tied it into bunches. We kept the tobacco hanging in his room for several weeks, but the dry atmosphere made the bunches continually crumble on the floor. I finally took one of the bunches and had it framed in a shadow box to hang on the gentleman's wall and it hung there until the day he died. When he passed away we moved the shadow box into the activity room for everyone to see.

We ended up with enough cucumbers with which to make dill pickles, so one day we set up an assembly line in the activity room and everybody had a job: washing the cucumbers, cutting the cucumbers, adding the dill and other ingredients, and packing the jars. When the jars were filled we took them to the kitchen to add the brine and process the pickles. Several weeks later we were eating of our patients' fruits of their labors.

We managed to get a couple of pumpkins to grow even though they were small ones, but we used them to decorate the facility during the fall. Several ladies were interested in collecting seeds for next year's garden, so we helped them do this by labeling paper bags with each name and sliding the seeds inside. The seeds were used the next spring, but many of the original patients were no longer around to see them be put in the ground.

We had one lady who didn't like to go outside but she grew the most beautiful African violets in her south-facing window. Her violets were so prolific that we had to have maintenance add a second shelf in the window to hold all her violets. She would start new ones from the leaves of the older ones and then baby them until they were big enough to grow unaided. It was always a joy to walk into her room and see all the beautiful violets blooming in every color imaginable.

These were just a few of the ways we tried to help transition patients into their new environments by trying to make them feel as much at home as possible. Although we provided activities every day, I must admit that gardening with these patients was the highlight of that summer. The local newspaper even came to do a story about the patients and their garden. Seeing their smiling faces and hearing them tell the reporters their story was so rewarding. This was one everyday activity we provided on a daily basis during growing season and it helped to make the patients feel like they were still contributing to society.

Elderly people enter nursing homes on a daily basis and it is the nursing staff's job to make these people feel as comfortable as possible. After doing a complete family history, many times it is easy to add new activities to someone's routine in order to make them feel needed and still in control of their lives. Continuing to work with the patients and their families is important as a means of keeping up-to-date with their needs, and it continues to keep them active and feeling alive.

Bobbi Dawn Rightmyer, Harrodsburg, April 12, 2012

MOTHER'S YEARS OF SERVICE

My mother was a native of Leslie County, born in 1900. When she decided to pursue a nursing career, she was not trained but was offered a position as maid in a Presbyterian family located in Philadelphia. So she worked as a maid at night but went to a nursing school at Chester County Hospital after she graduated from high school there in Philadelphia. She got her nursing training in Philadelphia through the Presbyterian Church.

The Frontier Nursing Service was not in Leslie County when my mother returned home as a nurse. My mother's sister had an eye infection and there was some type of public health clinic to which my mother took her when she was quite young. She was thinking that it was really neat to be a nurse. Mary Breckinridge was there about the time my mother returned, and the two of them rode around on horseback deciding where the hospital would be. I don't know what all transpired before then but these are some of the early memories of early things my mother had told me.

When my mother finished nursing school she was tops in her class, for which she got a gold five-dollar piece. At that point in time Mama's father was dying of typhoid fever back in Leslie County over on Hurricane [Creek]. She came back home, and she remembered placing that five-dollar gold piece in her dying father's hand. I think that impressed her to stay at home and [be] a nurse because that was also about the same time Mary Breckinridge came there. That was just a logical chain of events.

My mother did not like obstetrics but she liked surgery, so that's why she became Dr. Kooser's surgical nurse. She did some horseback riding as a nurse, and I remember her telling me about riding down the river with the doctor in order to amputate somebody's foot. I think it was a male patient who did not want the foot destroyed. Well, they buried the foot and he kept complaining several days later that his toes were hurting, so they dug up the foot and straightened the toes out and the man's pain went away. That was one of those weird things. I guess it was a sort of traditional mountain association about that type of thing. She wore a white uniform and did work in the hospital. She was never assigned to places like Redbird Clinic or any of the outposts.

By the time I was born my mother was no longer working at the hospital for the Frontier Nursing Service. At some point in time she decided to not continue that route, so she started a country store on Hurt's Creek, just up the road from our house. It was like a family company store for an opening coal mine. All mine employees had credit at the store in order to get groceries.

My mother was truly wonderful.

Told by Carrie M. Parker to Dale Deaton, September 29, 1979;
provided by the Louie B. Nunn Center for Oral History,
University of Kentucky Libraries, Lexington

Getting to Know Miss Breckinridge

While I was a junior courier in 1958 assisting in home deliveries, Miss Breckinridge had become a sort of matriarch of the Frontier Nursing Service. They were caring for her and she was viewed as the Queen Bee. She and Agnes Lewis would go up to her room on the second floor in the big house and do whatever was needed. She sat at the head of the table and Betty Lester sat at the far end and rang the bell when we needed something else removed or taken from the table. Yeah, she was truly the matriarch at that point.

At that point her vision was failing and she walked with a cane. We would gather the eggs, and she had this little basket she carried on one arm as we walked up to the chicken house to gather the eggs. She would always comment on how stupid chickens were, but yet they were some of her favorite creatures.

I can remember going up to have tea and to see her later on. When we walked over to her she would want to kiss you on the cheek, but we always had to tell her who we were. She always liked to give me a kiss.

Later on, two or three years before she died, she would sit in this one chair which nobody sat in and she would feed cubes of cheese to the dogs. She still liked to have you bend over so she could give you a little kiss. I think she died in 1966.

Told by Carrie M. Parker to Dale Deaton, September 29, 1979; provided by the Louie B. Nunn Center for Oral History, University of Kentucky Libraries, Lexington

Memories about Mary Breckinridge

I felt that Mrs. Breckinridge was a fairly easy person to talk to. I had several personal conversations with her, especially when this problem came up here and I had to sort of break my contract because I had signed up to go to Hyden, Kentucky. She was very easy to talk to, and I think sometimes people put her on a pedestal for a while until they realized she was really a down-to-earth person and lived her life just like the rest of us.

Living in the big house over at Wendover wasn't any different than living in the hospital or living in one of the centers. I think I always felt that she was very down-to-earth. Of course, she was the boss and you did what was necessary to carry out her directions. Nonetheless, I always thought she was very fair in the way she treated people.

I knew she was a very religious person and that the church was very important to her. We always had church services and she was there.

Told by Nancy N. Porter to Dale Deaton, March 5, 1979;
provided by the Louie B. Nunn Center for Oral History,
University of Kentucky Libraries, Lexington

INSPIRED BY MRS. BRECKINRIDGE

Mrs. Breckinridge went on speaking tours throughout the United States, and she was speaking in Cincinnati. At that point in time I had been doing some private duty nursing and I went out to hear her talk. She was really a character and a wonderful public speaker. So I heard her and was very intrigued, but it was very different from anything that I had done. So I wanted to take a vacation, but like many youngsters of that age I had very little money. So I asked Mrs. Breckinridge if I could volunteer for a month and ride horses in my off-duty hours. She said, "Yes, come on," then grabbed me.

I came on down here to Hyden and really fell in love with this place. I always loved to ride horses, so when I finished work in the afternoon I would take a ride for an hour and then be back to get the horse in the barn and be ready for dinner. I could also go riding after dinner.

Told by Grace Reeder to Carol Crowe-Carraco, January 25, 1979;
provided by the Louie B. Nunn Center for Oral History,
University of Kentucky Libraries, Lexington

FEELINGS OF THANKFULNESS

This is about a young lady whose name is Lenore and she was working at Wendover. Lenore was a beautiful, delightful child. She looked younger than she was. She had never finished high school but was exceedingly bright and was a wonderful musician. She could sing with her whole body and soul and did so as she sang.

I used to say to her, "Lenore, you should really try to get your high school education and get some tutoring so you can write your examinations. You would like to go into child care because you'd be very good with children."

Of course she didn't believe it until one day I caught her red-handed. I had an astrology book that had very big words in it. She'd come to my room every once in a while and say, for example, "Now, Trudy, could you [read it]?" Then she'd say, "Oh, that was interesting."

I'd say, "Okay, that means you can read and write."

She did go back to get her high school equivalency exam and has since graduated from college. Bright and sharp as a tack, but she didn't believe she had it. That same girl came to me one morning and said, "Trudy, may I ask you a question as to whether or not I am underprivileged?" She went on to tell me about how poor they had been and had to carry coal and water, but were happy and sang [together].

I said, "Well, as long as you were happy I don't think you should call yourself underprivileged. I think it's a very unfortunate word that crept into our language. But if you are happy I think you know best whether you're underprivileged or not."

She then said to me, "Thank you," while holding her head up high as she walked out the door. There are many other incidents of people who come and say, "I never felt underprivileged," because their young years were happy ones. The only way they felt they did not have as much as other people was due to lack of material things. Their relationships with other people and with other members of their family were typically rich ones. Basically you get it from people from every walk of life here in [Leslie and surrounding counties]. This was their lifestyle and they did not know anything else.

Compared with other persons, long ago you never knew who had money and who didn't.

Told by Gertrude Isaacs to Dale Deaton, November 15, 1978;
provided by the Louie B. Nunn Center for Oral History,
University of Kentucky Libraries, Lexington

SERVICE PAYMENTS

The Frontier Nursing Service never emphasized getting paid for anything. We treated anyone, no matter what, which I loved. I don't like not treating someone whom you know, but at some clinics you pay or else. I was concerned that some people had bills that ran for years and years and they'd never pay it off. I try to instill the principle, and this worked out with one young lady for whom I delivered several of her babies.

Most people didn't like not paying, even though some of them obviously didn't have the funds. Sometimes they'd try to pay in kind, like giving you fruits and produce and stuff like that, which is hard to write off on a bill. Some would pay off by doing work for so many hours. Most people didn't like not being able to pay.

We visited a prospective mother at least once a month if everything was normal. If they were lacking in something or needed more frequent blood work or were not well in some other way, we never waited for them to come [to the clinic]. If they missed one clinic appointment we went out after them. Many people in medical service feel that the patient should come and you shouldn't have to keep going after them.

On the home visits you got to know the families in the homes and what situations they were really in and why they didn't come [to clinics]. Maybe it wasn't their fault after all, due to the fact they had to walk five miles down a creek to get there or what was really going on in their home.

Most people we treated were wonderful and we were nice to them.

Told by Mary Penton to Dale Deaton, June 15, 1979;
provided by the Louie B. Nunn Center for Oral History,
University of Kentucky Libraries, Lexington

Resignation, but Not Yet

I once resigned from an emergency room eleven-to-seven nurse position that I loved. However, there were concerns I had that affected patient care and possibly my license and certainly my satisfaction [by] working there. I went ahead and resigned after providing a two months' notice, the latter due to the fact I knew I could not be easily replaced. Included with my resignation was a list of six things that needed to happen for the emergency room to be safe and functional.

A couple of weeks later the assistant nursing director came to talk with me and said, "We got your resignation."

I said I was making plans for leaving, and she responded by saying they got my note about the things I said needed changing and that they were going to do all of them, and then I asked her, "Who met relative to my resignation?" She responded by telling me it was the hospital administrator, the head of the various medical programs, nursing, and various heads of other departments. She added that they had already hired a medical director for the emergency room and he would be in to meet me the next morning.

We met and he went ahead to tell me he wanted me to stay awhile, as did the others, because they were going to do everything I had asked for.

I stayed several more years. My activities relative to resignation demonstrate that verbal suggestions can work but need to be followed by written summary and a thank-you for listening.

I want all registered nurses to know that they do have a voice, to be used not for complaining at lunch but being professional, and when you complain I think it is mandatory to offer the solutions that you believe are necessary for the well-being of the institution relative to dollars, reputation, and the best care for the patients, whose very lives depend on the hospital and its employees. Also, put your concerns in writing and send them even if you have presented your issues verbally.

Jeri R. White, Lexington, June 16, 2012

Mary Breckinridge Arrives in Leslie County

Mrs. Mary Breckinridge said in her book that my father and Judge C. Lewis were two of the first people she met in Hyden, and Father knew so much about her family. In fact she said Father knew more about her family than she did in some instances. He introduced her to the people in Leslie County, although she could make her own introductions. She had this friendly, warm way and people just accepted her immediately. And as you know, mountain people are not too ready to accept outsiders, since you have to prove yourself to them. But she was accepted very quickly there.

It was my happy privilege to ride with Mary a few times as she went out through the mountains and to talk to her on the trip. This is not history of Leslie County, but it is very personal. [My husband and I] had difficulty with the birth of our first child, and we still wanted more children. Mary said, "Oh, you go right on and have another baby. You come up here and we'll take care of you."

What she said gave me the confidence that I needed; thus our son Lewis, who is now fifty-two years old, was really born with the encouragement of Mary Breckinridge, and she always said that he was her baby! So I did know Mary there and, of course, my parents loved her dearly and had very, very happy association with her.

Mary's father came to Leslie County later and the first thing I heard about him was that he was so eager to do something helpful and constructive. After hearing that I thought it was the sweetest thing a man could do. He wanted some of the women who were good with a needle to teach the high school girls how to sew, and he then organized a little sewing club. That was one of the simplest things he could do but it was so valuable and it helped to show the greatness of the Breckinridge family. They had the ingenuity to see a need and to have the urge to fill it. He got some of the women there to come after school in afternoons to help [show] those young high school girls how to make buttonholes and how to sew a good seam and things like that. Nothing was too small or too great for the Breckinridges to undertake.

At the first meeting of Frontier Nursing Service, Mary told what she wanted to do in order to help the mothers and babies, to bring people in who could help in childbirth and in infant health and things like that. Of course, it was public health as much as maternal health that Frontier Nursing Service developed into.

She was well received and was a person who was so very acceptable, and her overflowing love for people, especially children, was bound to find response. Of course, the people then felt their personal needs in all stratas of life. As far as I know there was never any opposition. As previously stated, the mountain people do not accept outsiders readily, but as far as I know Mary was accepted wholeheartedly from the very beginning.

I was married in 1922, one year before she came, and then she was back in 1925, when the work on Frontier Nursing Service really began. My parents told me all about it, and they were closely associated with the FNS all the time.

Late one afternoon in late November, Mrs. Breckinridge rode over on her horse to see my mother. They lived over there on a hill opposite where the new Hyden Hospital is located. Mama went down to the gate to meet her at the foot of this little hill. Mrs. Breckinridge rode up and she and Mama were there talking. Mrs. Breckinridge looked upon the hill and saw the late afternoon sun on this chilly November afternoon shining on the point up there and she said, "Right there's where I want my hospital. Can I have it? Do you suppose I can get it?"

My mother said, "I'm sure you can because we own that land and my husband's nephew owns the adjoining land, so I'm sure you can have it."

Mary was impulsive, and when she saw the land for Wendover she said, "Someday I'm going to have me a house there," and sure enough, she did. She was a decisive person and never wasted time, which I thought was a great asset to the creative ability that she had. Then they got the stone there on the hill to build the hospital. Truth of the matter is, they split up the stone that I used to play on as a child, and I was glad to have it go into the hospital.

Told by Mary Lewis Biggerstaff, Berea, to Dale Deaton,
February 12, 1979; provided by the Louie B. Nunn Center
for Oral History, University of Kentucky Libraries, Lexington

MEMORIES ABOUT MARY BRECKINRIDGE

I have refrained from mentioning the death of Mary Breckinridge, and the grief of [the loss of] her children is a thing that has always touched me most deeply. I thought a great deal about Mary's motivation, which she had prior to her children. She was always one who could do things in order to meet the demands of her heart and her own mind. But the grief of her children has always touched me very deeply. There was something about Mary Breckinridge that drew out the best in people who knew her. She wasn't a person of piety or anything like that, but she had a great spirit to which people responded. I know our children always went so joyously when we'd go to her house. When Mary came bounding [up] the steps, the gentlemanly qualities our two little boys had came forth. They would always stand and meet her and bring out their best to honor her. It used to break my heart to see her stand and look, look, look at my children.

There was a deep spiritual motivation in all of her work. Her sister Adeline, who lived in England, had much spiritual influence on Mary's life and was such an influence on her work.

Told by Mary Lewis Biggerstaff, Berea, to Dale Deaton,
February 12, 1979; provided by the Louie B. Nunn Center
for Oral History, University of Kentucky Libraries, Lexington

LITTLE SHEPHERD BOY

This is a story told by Mary Breckinridge about a little boy that always played as an angel or something like that in the Christmas pageant. He always acted like an angel, perhaps because he was just a little kid who had got into his father's gristmill and had an accident that took away his arm. He was brought to the hospital and just shortly after, he woke up from anesthesia or something like that.

The nurse and his family gathered around and the little boy said to them, "Now I'll have to be a shepherd or something like that because they don't have to fold their hands."

I guess it was the Christmas pageant that was one of his first thoughts after the accident. He had always acted like an angel, and he folded his hands because they have to fold their hands. Mrs. Breckinridge thought what a wonderful, quick acceptance he portrayed after the loss of his arm.

The pageant that year was a real reward to me, since I was in a place where Christmas meant so much.

Told by Carolyn Booth Gregory, Evanston, IL, to Linda Green, March 31, 1979; provided by the Louie B. Nunn Center for Oral History, University of Kentucky Libraries, Lexington

AWARD-WINNING SERVICE

There was a male nursing student who cared for a prominent citizen in Elizabethtown. The way this student worked with this patient made a lasting impression on the family of the patient and they later established a scholarship for nursing students at Elizabethtown Community College because of that student and the care he had given to their family member.

I don't know whether the scholarship still exists or not, but it helped students out for several years.

Told by Martha Hill, Glendale, to Mark Brown, June 30, 2012; provided by the Kentucky Historical Society, Frankfort

SURPRISE BIRTHDAY CAKE

There was a sweet lady, Mrs. Throckmorton, who worked as a nurse's aide. At that time she was elderly to me. I'm not sure of her age, but I suspect she was at least sixty years old. On my birthday, November 1, 1961, I came to work and was given a huge surprise. After Mrs. Throckmorton had gotten off work the previous day she had baked me a cake. Once I got to work and while the doctors were making their rounds she gave me my birthday cake, which was a blackberry jam cake with caramel icing.

You talk about being good, I mean it was so delicious. Everyone enjoyed it and were able to go on to their work all the happier because of the kindness of Mrs. Throckmorton.

Evelyn Pearl Anderson, London, July 18, 2012

CANCER PATIENT'S BAPTISM

One of my most precious patient-related stories comes out of the hospital in Humansville, Missouri. During midafternoon I made my rounds and went to a very ill gentleman with terminal cancer who was being cared for by a private duty nurse. She told me that he had just accepted the Lord as savior and wanted to be baptized. A pastor had been called to come, and the question was raised as to where this man wanted to be baptized.

I went downstairs to the first floor behind the administrator's office, where the only full bathroom in the hospital was located. That is where the bathtub was located. I checked it carefully and found that there was only hot water available. Knowing what time to expect the pastor, I enlisted the help of one of the nurse's aides to locate a pail in which to carry cold water from the kitchen to the bathtub. While [we were] running the hot water and pouring the hand-carried cold water, the patient was being brought downstairs.

The pastor came and the patient was with his private duty nurse. I was with them at the bathtub and it was a very precarious situation because of the weight of the patient, his inability to move, and the level of pain he was having. I evaluated the situation and found a small step stool to place in the tub for the patient to sit on. I then took off my shoes and climbed into the tub. The three of us carefully lifted the patient into the tub, sitting him down on the step stool. It was from this position that the pastor was able to gently lower the patient into the baptismal waters as I supported the patient. The baptism was completed and the patient was then placed into a dry gown, after being thoroughly wiped with towels, and returned to his room.

Later I went to the room to administer some medication when his private duty nurse gave me five dollars. I told her I could not accept money, but she said, "Please take it. He wants you to have it because his baptism meant so much to him and giving it to you is all he can do."

I took the money. It was all I could do to reveal my true inspiration.

Evelyn Pearl Anderson, London, July 18, 2012

MISSION TRIP TO RUSSIA

This is about our 2007 Medical Missions trip by Eastern Kentucky Overseas Mission Team to a small village in Zlynka in southwestern

Russia near the Ukrainian border. We were up bright and early for breakfast during our trip to Zlynka and could peer past the old gray gate, and I could see people busily bringing tables outside and placing cloths on them. We were going to have an out-of-doors clinic. This was so exciting, even if the wind was blowing papers here and there. Patients were waiting to see us. The first thing on the agenda was to check out the toilet facilities. Our interpreters did that and soon we were seeing patients outside in the churchyard.

The church was in a house that some might think resembled an old chicken house. Nevertheless, the Christians were very proud of their church house. Inside the doorway, leaning against the wall, were two short brooms, handmade of sticks and tied with a cord. I showed such interest in them that Julia gave me one as she laughed. I am as proud of this Zlynka stick broom as a crystal dish from Dyatkovo.

We saw twenty-one persons in the clinic. The pastor, Piter, and his wife, along with members, brought out watermelon that they had saved from the Harvest Day worship service. Precious! We all did enjoy standing in the yard eating the melon and spitting the seeds, just like the old rural Kentucky way. After we finished we made two home visits.

The two home visits turned out to be clinics within themselves. The team got out of their van at the home of the patient. Dr. Jeff and I went in to see the young man, who had paralysis resulting from a stroke. While we were in the house five others wanted to be seen. The man's mother was a large lady with bronchial discomforts, and the man's wife was a diabetic, and their three little children were ill with respiratory problems. The home was poor with tiny rooms. The meager couches were used as beds. Apparently several persons slept in the tiny room. It looked as if the young mother and three children slept in one very small room.

I went out to the back of the van to get a trunk of medication in order to take in what was needed. The rest of the team helped the nurses get a trunk down on the street and assisted in finding the medications that were needed. When all six patients had been treated, the doctor and nurse joined two other team members who, with an interpreter, were across the street talking with several young and old men sitting on the bench. Before long those men began to tell Dr. Jeff their health problems. So he treated five persons on the street as they sat on the bench. The nurses and doctor ended up seeing thirty-two patients on that Tuesday.

A middle-age woman was standing there, and she looked at me, smiling, and said she wanted to say something. After a few minutes she said, "Alleluia." There we were on the street of Zlynka, a village where the Russian Orthodox threaten. I began singing the chorus, "Hallelu, hallelu, hallelu, hallelujah, praise ye the Lord."

The lady watched my lips closely and began trying to sing with me the second time around. By the third time, she had it down and sang loudly. There we were, a Russian lady and an American nurse loudly singing praises to the Lord on a street in Zlynka, a village written off by the government.

This was an incredibly wonderful experience that I shall never forget.

Evelyn Pearl Anderson, London, July 24, 2012;
revised September 28, 2013

CARETAKING THE DYING

One particular night a woman who was elderly, around ninety-four years of age, was on her deathbed and was under an oxygen tent. Sure enough, then the girls went in to check on her; they called me back and said to check her vital signs—there were none. Keep in mind that about thirty years ago we could let the elderly die in peace and dignity. I called her doctor and he came and pronounced her dead.

After the girls got her ready for the funeral home persons to come to get her, I went to check to see if she was ready. As I was walking down the hall, one of the CNAs [certified nursing assistant] came running out of the room, shouting, "She's not dead, she's not dead."

Well, I walked into the room and sure enough, after twenty minutes she started to breathe again. I ran to the nurses' station and called the doc, and that stunned him. He said, "If she doesn't stop breathing within twenty minutes or so, call me back again."

I didn't have to call him back because I stayed at her side and held her hand and talked with her, telling her that it was all right, that I was there. It wasn't long until she died peacefully.

Many times during my nursing career I have sat and held the elder's hand as they passed away, because they had no family, or the family didn't care.

Teresa Fryman Bell, Edmonson County, October 29, 2012

Nurses in Churches

Julie Dobernic, a nurse here in Bowling Green, doesn't take temperatures or apply Band-Aids. She doesn't work in a clinic or a hospital due to the fact the church is her doctor's office and prayer is her medicine. Eight years ago she hung up her hospital scrubs to become a nurse at Holy Spirit Catholic Church. She's part of a growing group of nurses who are taking positions within their religious institutions, and Western Kentucky University now offers a class on faith nursing.

The Faith Community Nursing class has been offered for the past six years and it's growing. Nearly fifty students took the class last academic year, and more nurses are specializing in church-based nursing at Western Kentucky University.

"We spend a lot of time having them to think about how they view health and what it means, and how the spiritual aspect impacts our health. . . . It's an online class, and has included students as far away as Alaska. Several students go on to become nurses in temples and mosques, but nearly all faith nurses in this area are part of Christian[ity]," according to Professor Siegrist. "But no matter the religion, nursing practices are similar," she said. "What makes it different from the hospital type of nursing is the nurse is very aware of the need to integrate body, mind, and spiritual needs. It's amazing the different types of things they do. In some cases, church nurses are paid, but many are not. Most area faith nurses are volunteers. . . .

"I think it's just really important for a church community and a faith community to support each other, to be there when times are tough."

From Jenna Mink, "Nurses in Churches,"
Bowling Green Daily News, *July 29, 2011*

Helping an Elderly Lady

Two events have sort of touched me that I was able to facilitate because you are who you are and where you are. I was working part-time and had come in to focus on my assignment that day, and it was to work on a ninety-two-year-old woman who was very ill and probably was not expected to live. I had her for about three days in a row, and when I left she was still not responding much, although we had gotten her up in a chair. And she was responding a little bit more.

I was off for a day, and when I came back she was just doing so well.

I was talking to her about how she was feeling and telling her how she looked. She said, "I know I was close to death and I saw all my brothers and sisters and they were waving to me to come on. But I then saw the Master and he told me I had to go back. I don't know why, and at ninety-two what would I possibly have to do?"

I said, "Well, you are obviously an inspiration for someone because you are still here." She was discharged and did very well for a number of years, because she was back in again when she was ninety-four or ninety-five. Then I happened to have her assigned as one of my patients for the day. So I went in and said to her, "I remember you."

She said, "I remember you, too, and for the life of me I can't understand why he sent me back." Then I thought how neat that was, because it really was a powerful event for me in developing my own understanding of death and dying. No matter what your religious beliefs are, or what your spiritual path is, being a part of a person's spiritual journey helps you to help others on their spiritual journey.

That was a profound event for me.

Patricia A. Slaten, Petersburg, March 6, 2013

STUDENT INSPIRATIONAL EVENT

As I grew up in Letcher and Perry Counties in eastern Kentucky, I heard many stories about Mary Breckinridge and her Frontier Nursing Services nurses. I was fascinated by the stories of their riding horseback to take care of their patients. By the time I went to Berea College for my nursing education, Mary Breckinridge was elderly but was still living in Hyden at the Frontier Nursing Service.

Frances Allen, our public health instructor, took my class on a field trip to Frontier Nursing Service to meet Mary Breckinridge. My memory of her is that she was sitting on the front porch smoking a cigarette using a long, skinny cigarette holder. She said to us, "I hope you girls are not smokers because it is not good for you. At my age, this is the only vice I can handle."

She took time to talk with us about our nursing studies. She said, "You know there are times when I worry about the state of nursing in our country, but when I meet you young nurses, I know that nursing is going to be all right." This statement really impacted me emotionally.

Clara Fay Smith, Erlanger, March 6, 2013

Fulfilling Request of a Dying Woman

I was working on a Sunday, a day that is typically less hectic than some other days of the week. I was talking with one of my patients, a young woman in her midforties who was in the last days of her life as a result of cancer. She was alert and knew what was going on. [I was] asking her if there was anything she would like for lunch or anything at all to eat, and her reply was, "I would love to have a big McDonald's with french fries before I die."

Since we were not allowed to leave the hospital, I was confronted with a decision: to either break the rules or deny her request. I broke the rules and sent an aide to the town for a Big Mac and fries. Fortunately all proceeded well and we didn't get caught, but I really didn't care.

The lady ate very little, but that was expected. It wasn't how much she ate but that she had the opportunity to eat it. Unfortunately, she died about four days later. The staff felt good about what we had done.

Patricia A. Slater, Petersburg, March 6, 2013

Youthful Inspiration to Be a Nurse

When I was in the sixth grade in the Flemingsburg Elementary School I was asked to be the nurse in a class play. How exciting! My friend and sixth-grade classmate, Dorothy, had an older half-sister, Mauvereen, who was a registered nurse but had died early in life. Dorothy's family let me borrow Mauvereen's nurse cap for the play. I remember being on "cloud nine" with the cap pinned onto my hair, but I don't know how I did in the play. I think that surely [the] dome of my excitement must have shown forth.

When I became sixteen I dedicated my life to the Lord as a missionary nurse in a worship service in the Flemingsburg Methodist Episcopal Church South. Of course, I was still in high school, but I KNEW what I was going to do.

During my junior year of high school I entered the Fleming County Farm Bureau King-Queen Contest. There was a time for a public interview during the contest, and the question was asked, "What are you going to do?" No one was surprised when I said, "Be a nurse."

The next question was, "Where are you going to school?" I told them it was the St. Joseph Hospital School of Nursing in Lexington,

Kentucky. My parents were shocked because everyone knew I was planning to attend Good Samaritan Hospital School of Nursing in Lexington, which was supported by the Methodist denomination. . . . The day came in August 1957 when my father drove me to Lexington, accompanied by my mother, brother, and sister. Lexington was about sixty miles southwest of Flemingsburg, seemingly very far away. There I entered the Good Samaritan Hospital School of Nursing.

The family left and I was in a brand-new environment with my dream before me, a family foundation under me, a bountiful faith over me, but little knowledge of the world ahead of me. However, I was really excited, and it was there I began studying to become a nurse.

Evelyn Pearl Anderson, London, July 18, 2012

WONDERFUL MEMORIES OF SERVICE

My first nursing job was on a med-surge floor, and I loved it and stayed there for three years. My most memorable patients included one frequent flyer who was an alcoholic with COPD [chronic obstructive pulmonary disease]. He had a sad background due to the fact his brother was also his father, thus he was not 100 percent mentally there. However, he would come in completely dehydrated and coughing profusely after smoking too much. Then the task would be to prevent him from leaving the floor attached to his IV pole, since he would run away across the street to the bar and drink beer, and then the police would have to bring him back.

Another memorable patient was the man in his forties who had never been sick a day in his life. He worked on a farm raising cattle. One day he accidentally got gored by one of his bulls and had a huge gash in his stomach. Any normal person would think that would involve a trip to the ER. However, as the man had never succumbed to any sickness before in his life, he simply asked his wife to sew him up, and she kindly obliged, since she was used to sewing up the cows after they gave birth or had any kind of injury.

Naturally the poor man came in with a raging infection and required wound debridement surgery.

When he went home he told us he was going to name his two new calves after the doctor who did the surgery and after me, the nurse who looked after him. I was very flattered, as I had never had a cow named after me before that.

I remember the man who came in with multiple fractures after he laid on top of his wife and their child in a bathtub when a tornado ripped through his house.

I also remember the lady who came in with breast cancer, which rapidly progressed into vena cava syndrome, where she could not lie down since she could not breathe if she did. I remember her so well because even though she was so sick and going for emergency radiation treatment, when I walked into her room I saw that she had put on some crazy eyeglasses with fake eyeballs hanging out on springs. She was trying to joke with me despite her grave situation.

I never found out what happened to her; such is the nature of hospital shift nursing, sometimes on for three days in a row and off work for four days. Then when you come back and there were a whole new array of patients there.

Being involved with all these nice people as their nursing servant is partly what inspired me to go back to school to get my master's degree and become a nurse practitioner. I wanted to work in an office with the same flow of patients coming back on a regular basis and really get to follow a patient's health throughout their life course. So for three long years I sometimes questioned myself as to why I went back to school.

I have now survived the first year of being a nurse practitioner and am incredibly thankful that I wake up every day and love my job. It has been a very steep learning curve and it is very challenging, but I love how every day is different.

The Forest Gump adage of "Life is like a box of chocolates, you never know what you're going to get" is a definite mantra for involvement in health care.

Louise Webb, Bowling Green, June 10, 2013

Rationale for Loving Patients

Favorite patients that I have now come to love and know include a man with just 15 percent of his lung function left. He has been on the lung-transplant list for seven years. The fact that he has struggled for his every breath for the past seven years is unimaginable, as most of us take breathing as a natural given, something automatic that requires no thought from us. For him it is a constant effort every waking minute.

I love his wife too due to the dedication and tireless worry for her husband that she shows.

I have also grown to love our frequent flyer, who is a highly anxious lady who will come and see me every week complaining that she just cannot swallow. She has had every scope, tube, and light thrust down her throat by several doctors and swallow studies galore, all indicating the likely cause of dysphagia [difficulty swallowing] as being psychogenic, or [due to] extreme anxiety. So we give her a high five when she proudly comes to tell us she has managed to eat Cheetos earlier this week, and we patiently educate her each time she comes about her problems.

We all love to see our favorite patients. We probably shouldn't have favorites, but we can't help it, especially when they bring us homemade cherry pies and brownies, or freshly grown corn or tomatoes from their gardens.

Louise Webb, Bowling Green, June 10, 2013

READY TO DIE AND GO TO HEAVEN

Recently, after hanging up my stethoscope thinking my nursing experiences were over, I had one more event. A dear friend's mother, at the age of ninety-five, a resident in a nursing home, started to say she was ready to die and go to heaven. She said that to everybody, including the nursing staff. She told the new preacher on his first visit to see her; she told her doctor and told it to all of her daughters.

This went on for days, weeks, and months. Her health would decline and then miraculously improve time and time again. Confusion was her most common symptom.

One afternoon when my friend went to visit her mother she found her mother trying desperately to undress herself. My friend tried everything to persuade her mom to keep her clothes on her body. Finally, frustration overwhelmed her and she asked her mom what she was trying to do. Her mom said, "I told you! I am ready to go to heaven and see Jesus"; then she went on to say, "I came into this world naked and I need to be naked to leave it!"

My sweet friend, with tears in her eyes, told her mom that when Jesus came to get her he would bring her a brand-new gleaming white gown, and until then she needed to keep on her earthly gown. It worked! And it worked time and time again when confusion made her restless and the gown fidgeting began.

Well, her wait shortly came to an end. Very early one morning Jesus did come to get her. From the lasting smile on her face, he must have brought her the most beautiful heavenly gown she had ever seen!

Theresa Sue Milburn King, Danville, June 18, 2013

7

Nursing Training and Career Memories

Stories in this chapter describe numerous reasons for acquiring a nursing education and how individual nurses moved along with their career activities. Most anticipated that they would earn a nice salary, but they also wanted to help patients in need of serious, dedicated services.

Numerous nurses describe their work teaching in nurse-training schools. While most students were highly interested in earning good grades so as to obtain good jobs, some lost interest during the educational process. Some women talk about feeling the need for nurse training so as to properly raise their own children.

The bulk of the stories in this chapter, however, describe the routine work of nurses, such as giving a patient a final bath, delivering babies, teaching and working with midwives, or taking children to a neighbor's house in order to allow their mother privacy during the delivery of a baby, as well as deaths and burials.

Keynote Address to Other Nurses

When Kay Heady called to invite me to share my story at this annual luncheon of community health nurses, May 11, 2010, I said, "What an honor to be invited to speak to a group of community health nurses! Stand up and I will tell you why I think this is an honor. It is an honor because community health nurses are the salt of the earth, the sun in the sky, rain that washes away unwanted dust, and the rainbow that breaks forth after the storm."

As I reflected on my nursing background and journey I learned it was difficult to totally separate my life journey from my nursing story. The truth is that our nursing stories intertwine with the life we live; that includes where and to whom we were born, how we lived, and how we learned to interpret life events, and [it] shape[s] who we are as nurses today. So I'll begin with my early voices that continue to lie at the center of my heart.

First, I am a Kentuckian, born in a small town called Morganfield. I love Kentucky, but as an adult I traveled and searched for a more magical place to live. However, the more I traveled, the more I knew that Kentucky, with all its faults, was the place I dearly loved and the place I wanted to be.

Second, I am a farmer. When I was six years old my father, mother, and four siblings moved to a farm in Waverly, Kentucky. . . . My grandfather, who was orphaned when he was thirteen, traveled to Morganfield and became a wealthy man during the war [World War II], when his small cleaning and pressing shop was the only place in town for the nearby Camp Breckinridge soldiers. . . . Because of the land we owned we were considered among the wealthy in our small communities, but wealthy farmers had no money and no things that gave them status. . . . Wealth meant good weather, nourishing food, and friends who joined together in gatherings during the bad weather that stole the fruits of our work. Entertainment was what we could creatively imagine and do where we lived, and I can tell you that my friends imagined a lot!

On the farm I learned the celebration of birth in the spring and acceptance of death that inevitably came. From my grandparents, who were good and honest people, . . . I learned what life could and should be. Their steady values and commitment were planted in my being and carried me through life. Early on, I knew I had to be a healer. I know that for as long as I can remember the feeling was always there. When I saw a person or animal in pain I knew I had to stay until we could heal or bless the life that was fading. I wonder if there is a genetic influence that selects us as nurses, physicians, and other healers. From the Sisters of Charity of Nazareth who taught me for twelve years at St. Vincent Academy I learned that all life is precious, all life deserves respect, and that we are our brothers' and sisters' keeper. . . .

Rural Kentucky was a good place to live as a child or teen, but once past that time the opportunities were few. . . . My mother believed women should not work. I thought about going to a secretarial school in Evansville, but the bishop told my parents I would go to hell because it was not a Catholic school. Ready to move on with life, at almost eighteen years old I married a man seven years older than that. . . .

In high school I worked in a drugstore each day after school; then after I married in 1958 I began working as a lab assistant at Morganfield

Hospital, and in about a year I became a nursing assistant. What an experience that was! There were only two physicians in town and those of us left in the hospital had to figure a lot of things out. I did everything, including giving ether to woman who were in labor. Ignorance is bliss, or more realistically, a risk for the patient.

Later I moved with my husband to Henderson and was hired as a lab/office assistant for an internal medicine physician. I loved working there, as I grew my knowledge of many things. . . . The opening of Henderson Community College in the 1960s provided opportunities that changed my life and many others'. . . . In 1965, at age twenty-five, I entered college there just to take one class, so I thought. . . . During the first nursing lecture our instructor taught us three guiding principles and continued to do that [repeat them] at every opportunity during the program. The three guiding principles are: all persons have worth and dignity, all persons deserve to be treated with respect and care, and when immediate needs are met more mature needs emerge. . . . As nurses, I hope you will reach out with strong and steady hands to individuals like me and help them take that first, small step.

After graduation from Henderson Community College I worked at Methodist Hospital as an RN and simultaneously began taking the first next class for the new AD-BSN [associate to bachelor of science in nursing degree] program at the University of Evansville. It was during this time I learned community health. We had a powerful community health nursing faculty [member], Dorothy Hausman. She lived, ate, and breathed community health. Early on, she opened a nursing clinic in an underserved area and walked the streets giving the people things they needed. Our community health nursing course consumed us the entire semester.

There was no strategic long-term career planning. Committed first to our families, my generation of nurses perceived that we were place bound. We systematically decreased barriers to our personal and professional status and opportunistically took advantage of programs we created or access that we had demanded. Nurses were woman and liberation became our agenda in almost all areas of our lives.

The rewards were great. While at the University of Evansville my children and I were exposed to and gained from a private liberal arts college with a mission to facilitate the development of whole, healthy, happy, and educated persons who would graduate successfully and go forth to live the life they personally designed. As a part of my teaching assignment, we lived for three months in a castle at Harlaxton Manor in Grantham, England, on a four-day teaching assignment with travel strongly encouraged during the remaining three days.

I taught community health nursing while there but, of course, I learned more than I taught. I started a health service at the manor for the college students. When I arrived at Harlaxton, students who were sick would go to the house dame, who would give them medications. When I arrived I was given the charge of starting a health clinic. As I was preparing a clinic I looked for available medications, and I found that the popular house dame was giving the student[s] opium. No wonder why the students loved her!

During the 1970s gerontology became a national focus. The dean sent me to the first conference [of the] Association of Gerontology in Higher Education and subsequently to the first summer session on aging at the University of Hawaii in Honolulu. Thereafter I developed a multidisciplinary gerontology center, a nursing specialization, and a multidisciplinary certificate in aging. In doing this I learned the value of the community-based social worker, music therapist, and others. I learned the right question was not who was best to lead the team but rather, how could we work as a team to help the patient? Funded by the Southwestern Regional Council on Aging, I also developed a mobile health center for older Americans, staffed by a nurse practitioner that traveled through six rural counties. I received a Midwest Nursing Achievement Award for improving the health of older Americans. It amazes me that thirty-plus years later, nurse practitioners still have to fight for the right to bring the quality skills they possess to patients in need.

In 1986 I accepted a faculty position at the University of Louisville. My sons were off to another college and the free tuition at the University of Evansville was no longer needed. I was recruited as a gerontological nurse. I never lost my love for nursing practice, so throughout my academic career I practiced nursing part-time. . . . History repeats itself, and once again, when the education was complete, I set about developing and administering a family nurse practitioner program at the ULSON [University of Louisville School of Nursing].

In 2000 I received a call from Martha Dawson, nursing director at University of Louisville Hospital, who told me about the new building the Presbyterian Community Center in Louisville was going to build. She asked me if I would help start nursing programs there. Our plan was to put an NP [nurse practitioner] in the community center under the direction of the community center, but the lack of anyone with health expertise left the program floundering. Hence, in 2003 the program was moved to the University of Louisville's School of Nursing. We saw the opportunity to place nurses where they could practice nursing in its truest form. . . . With the expertise of [numerous nurses, some of whom were from the health department], nursing students, as well as physician colleagues, we came a long way in developing and implementing several dynamic programs. . . .

In closing, my five closing remarks are my take-home messages for you:

First, the choices I made were shaped by the choices I had, given the limited knowledge I had. We need to help others see farther than I can see.

Second, my career path was opportunistic. Although the ideal may be to have the broader plan at the beginning, if other options are not available, being opportunistic is a viable way to begin. We can help others see that a small first step is often the most important step. How does one eat an elephant? Simply one bite at a time!

Third, I am thankful for the wise persons who eased academic barriers that allowed me to pursue higher education. Our goal should be to continue to remove all barriers that limit the potential of under-served persons.

Fourth, I want nurses to demonstrate the strong leadership that shaped early nursing while keeping their focus on people. I hope for a sustainable community nursing model that puts nurses in leadership roles so they are free to be the nurses they are educated to be and [to] make the difference of which they are capable.

Fifth and finally, I am grateful to be a nurse where, during every day, the work has meaning and purpose. I am grateful to be counted among those who make up the most trusted profession. Enjoy this precious profession and keep it great by always keeping the patient or client at the center of your practice.

Dr. Kay T. Roberts, Louisville, December 17, 2011

UNANTICIPATED WISDOM FROM AN UNLIKELY SOURCE

This is a nursing tale of an unexpected lesson I learned from an unlikely teacher. It shaped my vision of nursing education. I was a young nurse faculty member about age thirty, teaching a medical-surgical course with a team of six nursing faculty members. Nursing students took this course during the second year of a four-year nursing program. The course was the right place for me. The course content focused on diseases. I, and most of us in the course, believed that health was a physical matter. Find the disease, give the right medicine, cut the pathogen out when needed, shape a healing environment, and health would appear. I was known as a "walking Guyton" and was named this because I knew just about every fact in the nine-hundred-page pathophysiology course textbook, authored by Guyton. I wanted to be the best nurse that one could be, and I believed that knowing these physical facts was essential. Students should also be able to excel, not just pass, in every aspect of the health program.

Each member of my faculty had a group of students, usually about six, whom they supervised during the sixteen-week clinical experience and in the theory portion of the course. All faculty members participated in teaching the theory lectures, and lectures were all there were. Requirements for passing the course were high. Students not only had to excel on the clinical unit, they had to pass the course with a B+ or A-level grade.

We were under pressure from faculty at the junior and senior levels of the program in order to pass capable students. On relatively rare occasions students failed a course during the third or fourth year of the nursing program. When this happened my nursing team was blamed for not eliminating students who could not "make it" in the program, thereby causing the students unnecessary loss of time and money, and costing the senior-level faculty grief and precious time. Also, in the early years students could not return to the nursing program if they failed a course. Later they could petition but were only allowed to reenter the program if all faculty agreed. So when a student failed in their junior or senior year, they failed the nursing program. It was a serious dilemma.

To help students, I often tutored those who were struggling [with] the exams on a one-on-one basis. I met with them to review questions they scored wrongly, coached them on how to study, and sometimes retaught content. A couple of these students subsequently failed at the next level of their nursing education, and eventually I vowed to be more discriminating in selecting students to tutor.

About this time one of the students in my clinical group barely passed her theory exam. I called her in and talked with her about her exam score. I asked her how I could help. She conveyed to me that she just could not get interested in all this "physical" stuff. I advised her that they [the school] may want to consider dropping [her from] the program on the possibility that she might fail at a higher level if she could not do well in our course. She thanked me and subsequently passed the course, but barely. Surprisingly, she began to flourish during her senior year when she entered the community health nursing course.

Five years after she graduated I picked up the local newspaper and there was her picture on the front page. There was a story of her amazing contributions to the health of a local community. She had become an established, successful, effective community health nurse leader, despite the fact that she was not very good with medical-surgical nursing.

The account awakened me, and I revisited major assumptions I had made about nursing education and the basic knowledge all nurses need. I became more aware that nursing is truly a varied profession, with many hating nursing. The community was where this nurse belonged. The community was where she was competent and dynamic. This led me to realize that it is nursing educators' charge to recognize and support unique strengths of the nursing students. Subsequently, I began to analyze unique characteristics of individual students and how these characteristics should influence the established curriculum. I learned that students teach as well as faculty. I began the transition from a novice faculty to an experienced faculty. I had learned an important lesson.

Dr. Kay T. Roberts, Louisville, January 29, 2012

CHOOSING TO BECOME A NURSE

As a divorced mother of two children, I decided to take my mother's advice and go to college to be a nurse. I was not sure if I wanted to become a nurse, but there was a nursing shortage and the pay was more than I ever dreamed of.

Katherine Catlett of the Bluegrass Community Action Center was an angel on earth when it came to me going back to school. She was kind and caring and understood the fact I needed to increase my education in order to raise my children the way I wanted them to be raised. It was Katherine who encouraged me to get my registered nursing degree instead of just a licensed practical nursing degree. The cons to this plan were another extra year of school, but the pros were a significant increase in pay. In 1987 registered nurses were being paid $9.50 an hour and there was a huge need. I could get a job anywhere I wanted.

The first thing Katherine had me to do was sign up for food stamps, but I had to put that off due to pride, even though I qualified. Katherine told me to start thinking about my children and not my pride, and that was the push I needed to sign up. The food stamps would help stretch my eighty-dollars-a-week child support payment, since my Pizza Hut salary, where I worked, would be decreased with me going to school full time.

The next thing Katherine helped me do was get out of the tiny two-bedroom apartment I was in and into a tiny two-bedroom Housing and Urban Development (HUD) house, partially paid by the government. My rent was eighty dollars a month, which was going to help with my cost of living, even though I still had electric, water, and garbage utilities to pay. The decrease in rent would be helpful.

While I was moving myself and the girls into our new house, Katherine was busy finding every grant and scholarship available in order to help me to go to nursing school. Pell Grants and nontraditional student scholarships were all strange to me. I was married when I was still in high school, so I had paid no attention to all the college information the guidance counselor handed out. Why did I need to go to college when I was married? I thought all the college kids were just wasting their time and that their hindsight was really twenty-twenty.

When August 1987 rolled around, my daughter Marie was enrolled in Head Start and rode the bus to school every day. Amber, my other daughter, was starting kindergarten and rode in a carpool from the day care center. We all three started school at the same time—Head Start, Harrodsburg kindergarten, and Midway College. My life had made a complete 180-degree turn. School was hard. I had been a straight-A student in high school, but I was not prepared for college and the different types of learning and testing, not to mention the endless papers that had to be written. Because I had not taken college courses in high school, my first year at Midway was basic introductory work for any incoming freshmen, even if I were twenty-five years old. I learned very quickly that I was not the only nontraditional student; thus several of us grouped up and helped each other through the grueling three years it took to get our nursing degree.

I would get home in the afternoon about the time Amber was getting home from school, but Marie would have been at the day care for just over two hours by the time I could pick the girls up. Home we would go, with an occasional stop at the park if the weather was pretty. I missed being able to spend time with my girls, so I tried to make up for it whenever possible. When we would get home it would be supper time. I tried to plan ahead what I was going to fix for supper every morning as we were wolfing down our breakfast.

After supper it was homework time. Marie didn't have homework, but I was surprised at the amount of homework Amber had, since she was only five years old. There were also my tons and tons of homework. Since my new boyfriend, Keith Rightmyer, and I had been dating for less than a year, he would come over after supper and help keep the girls entertained so I could get my homework done. He bought me my first typewriter, and that made writing papers so much easier.

For three years we followed this same routine—school, playtime, supper, work, homework, playtime, and then to bed. Many of my nights were complicated by my continuing to work part-time at the Pizza Hut. I wanted to show my daughters it was possible to raise a family and go to school and work at the same time. When I started my nursing classes I quit the Pizza Hut and began working as a certified nursing assistant at Ephraim McDowell Regional Medical Center in Danville, Kentucky. I typically worked a twelve-hour shift on Saturday and Sunday, so that cut into my time with my girls. Again, Keith was my hero and would babysit on the weekends when the girls were not at their father's house.

One of the proudest days of my life was when my parents, Bobby Gene and Brenda Sallee, my eight- and ten-year-old daughters, my grandmother Lura B. Sallee, and my new fiancé (Keith) attended my graduation from Midway College, 1990, and my pinning ceremony as a registered nurse (ADN [associate's degree in nursing]). The next week I remarried and began work as a fledgling RN studying for my state board examination.

All the foregoing accounts show that when one door closes, many more open.

Bobbi Dawn Rightmyer, Harrodsburg, February 22, 2012

Nursing Education

I entered the three-year diploma nursing program at Murray State University one week prior to my seventeenth birthday. We were required to complete two semesters at Murray, spend the following summer at a hospital for clinical rotation, then return to Murray for another semester.

At Murray we took general education courses along with biology, anatomy, physiology, chemistry, nutrition, bacteriology, psychology, and basic nursing courses. We received about fifty-six [credit] hours during three semesters. It was tough, but we managed to have fun also. In anatomy and physiology we were required to dissect a cat. The lab was right before lunch, and we had a great time discussing what we had done in the lab while eating at the table with friends who were not majoring in nursing. Come to think about it, we lost a few friends that semester.

Getting the experience at Murray before going to the hospital was a good thing. I was young, naïve, and ignorant about the ways of the world. I did a lot of "growing up" before I had to experience the world of medicine, and the world of medicine was what spared my ignorance for a while.

Ruth A. Buzzard, Dawson Springs, February 23, 2012

TICKS AT SCHOOL

My supervisor gingerly laid the phone back in the cradle and peered at me sideways over the glasses perched on the end of her nose. As a new school health nurse in the county, I had been filling out the endless forms when she had taken the call. "Well, it looks like it is time for you to go to work," she said to me. "You can finish those papers later."

"What's going on?" I asked her.

"Lice," she answered. "We're going to check students' heads." Yuck, I thought, itchy, crawly things on little people.

As we drove to the elementary school I flashed back in my mind to images of a girl in my sixth-grade [class] who wore a turban to school after her mother suddenly cut her [hair] real short. The girl was not happy about this. Naturally shy and rumored to be quite poor, her younger brother had also gotten a "butch" at the same time. But my school was small, with no sports for girls, and I hadn't attended a sleepover yet. I don't recall where we hung our coats. Anyway, nobody checked our heads, and I hadn't seen "nits" or their parents before this day.

There were three fourth grades and we were to check them all. I was shown what to look for, which were translucent white eggs— "nits"—glued to hair shafts at back of neck and behind ears. Soon I was mesmerized by different textures and patterns on these children. My supervisor sat in a chair, with children coming to her in a moving line. Her deft, experienced fingers moved quickly over their heads as she spoke to them about not sharing hats, combs, brushes, etc. Half-watching her to learn, I bent over each child and examined closely, getting a kink in my back before long.

And then there it was, something very strange indeed. Parting short, stiff, vanilla-colored hair, we found a one-centimeter blue/red raised button on the back of a boy's head. "Holy cow," I hissed to her, "what is that?"

"Oh Lord," she moaned. "It's a tick!"

A tick?!! What in the heck is that? My mother and her brother were not allowed to have pets during the cash-strapped times of the Great Depression and real estate speculation in Florida. As a result, she forbade the same in my childhood home. Except for one short-lived stint with an unfortunate puppy when I was in the fourth grade and a cocker spaniel next door that barely left the house, my experience with dogs was pretty limited. Oh, I had spent time in the woods as an adult, some of it with my friends and their dogs. Of course, I knew about fleas, since they made dogs scratch and were famous in circuses perhaps. But I had never seen a button-like thing attached to the back of somebody's head! What was this job going to entail?

I was soon to find out, as my supervisor sequestered the host child and fished in her purse for her matchbook. "Ask the teacher if she has tweezers," she ordered me, which sent the harried woman looking through a drawer that contained everything from confiscated gum to extra shoelaces. Producing the instrument, then the teacher gave the class a difficult assignment to divert their curious attention while she brought the four of us (one child, two school health nurses, and the tick) to a place with the best light.

The child didn't seem too upset about all this, thus causing me to wonder if he'd been through this before. My supervisor moved with quick assuredness while instructing me in ways of treatment. After cleansing the site with alcohol and with me holding the short stubble of hair away, she held a lit match near the tick for just a second in order to make it retreat a little. Then she firmly grasped the swollen creature with the tweezers and gently pulled. Well, there it was, a complete extraction! Swiping the area with the alcohol once more, she gave the boy a hug and sent him back to his seat.

We couldn't talk about the incident too much just then because there were a lot more heads to check for lice and nits. But it stayed with me for a long time and changed my behavior for a while.

I got real paranoid walking under trees that touched my hair and always checked my socks or pant cuffs after I'd been in the woods or brush. Sometimes I'd find one and brush it off with a little shiver of fright. My hand would then involuntarily go to the back of my head to see if a good climber had established a dinner table in the locks above my neck.

Then one day I went hiking during the late spring. I had on short pants and sat down on some rocks at one point. Later that night I found an attached tick on the inside of my thigh. Yikes! I practically jumped around the room. I was alone and matchless. Shaking, I rambled through my travel bag and thankfully found some tweezers. Then I recalled some of the other nurses saying if you didn't keep those tweezers around all of it, the head would stay embedded. I couldn't think about that! Just get it out! As I applied the instrument as I had seen my supervisor do, I became immediately calm. The tick came out intact.

"Huh," I said aloud. "That was nothing."

Terry Foody, LaGrange, March 12, 2012

PATIENT'S FINAL BATH

One of the first patients that I took care of as a student nurse had cancer with a short life expectancy. When I walked into his hospital room at 7:00 a.m. he was lying in liquid feces. I asked him if he were ready for a bath, and he said, "Let's let the washing slide."

I told him he would feel better after a bath. I washed him from one end to the other, and he went to sleep.

When I came back to clinical service a few days later I found out that he had died. At least he died clean.

Jo Ann M. Wever, Springfield, March 14, 2012

SURPRISED BY PATIENT'S IDENTITY

During a clinical rotation my instructor gave me an older female patient to take care of. When I walked into the patient's room I recognized her. She had been the professor who taught me an English course. I came out of the room and announced to my nursing instructor that my patient had been my English instructor.

My nursing instructor got pale and asked how I had done in the class. When I told her that I had made an A, she relaxed and breathed a sigh of relief. I always wondered what she would have done if I had told her that I flunked the course!

Jo Ann M. Wever, Springfield, March 14, 2012

NURSING THROUGH THE YEARS

I have the pleasure of being a former registered nurse. I was a non-traditional student, putting myself through nursing school as a single mother of two young children under the age of five years old. A question came to my mind recently when I was writing my first book, *Images of America: Harrodsburg.* The question was, how did we get a hospital in Harrodsburg, Kentucky? [Harrodsburg] being a city of firsts, I set out on a quest to find the answer to this question.

Some younger citizens will be surprised to hear there have actually been three hospitals in Harrodsburg, and the history reveals the great influence that women had in this wonderful history.

The women's club opened the first hospital on North Greenville Street by using a capital amount of $850 and renting a house. This property is now part of the Spring Hill Cemetery. That was such a wonderful example of female leadership. Where did they find a trained nurse (RN) to hire? How much did they pay her? What hours did she work? What medical cases were admitted? Did she deliver babies, serve the emergency room patients, cook food? And just how did her work day go? The early telephone operators worked twenty hours and then slept on a couch to take calls coming in during the next four hours. Is that how the "trained nurse" did it?

I have had to do a little speculation based on what little information I could find, and the answer is that she probably did a little of it all based on the needs. No doubt there were hot compresses to put on wounds and infections, cold sponge baths for the feverish, some laudanum for pain, perhaps some castor oil for the unfortunate impacted, and tincture of belladonna for dyspepsia. Did she have a thermometer or just the touch of the back of her hand on the patient's forehead?

It would be wonderful if someone would call me up and say, "Hey, Bobbi, I have my grandmother's handwritten journal that will answer some of your questions." What an awesome find that would be for me and for the history of Harrodsburg. I recently read an oral history interview recorded in 1990 from a lady who told about one of her experiences at the A. D. Price Memorial Hospital around 1948. A. D. Price Memorial was the second hospital in Harrodsburg. This lady talked about going there for her confinement and delivery of her baby girl. Her doctor came and examined her and went home after telling the nurse, "Call me when she's ready to deliver." Well, he should have stayed right there, because the nurse ended up delivering the baby. This happened to me a number of times when I was working night shift as a labor and delivery nurse.

I also talked with a night-shift nurse that everyone in the community just loved. She had to run up and down the stairs, and the employees and some patients would laugh about hearing the steps "speaking," but they never knew if this nurse were coming or going.

That reminded me of my own experience as a student nurse at Ephraim McDowell Regional Medical Center in Danville, 1987–1990. The nurses used the students like "go-fers," and we were not allowed to use the elevators. I worked on the sixth floor, and believe me, after a dozen or more trips up and down those stairs my tail would be dragging at the end of my shifts.

I can still remember giving cold or ice baths to reduce elevated temperatures, but we also had fever-reducing acetaminophen. We did have injectable painkillers like morphine and Demerol, but these became much easier to give with the use [of] intravenous lines. I remember the community bottle of alcohol and cotton balls for everyone's use, but now we have individual, wrapped cotton swabs. I can also remember not wearing gloves to start intravenous lines or draw blood work. Nowadays gloves are a must in every hospital procedure, not only to protect yourself but also to protect your patients. I can remember mixing our own intravenous fluids right in the nursing station. This is a big no-no today, since the pharmacy mixes all the fluids and special medications.

I completed my registered nurse training in 1990 and immediately went to work on the labor and delivery unit at Ephraim McDowell. I worked night shift there for almost fifteen years before transferring to the James B. Haggin Memorial Hospital in Harrodsburg. I had come home to my own community. Haggin Hospital is the third hospital we have seen in Harrodsburg. It was built on the grounds of the old Graham Springs Spa area, where people in the early 1800s would come to take the mineral waters.

I retired from nursing in 2005 after the death of my younger sister. I just did not have the spark to continue on with my nursing career. My goal had been to get a job and raise my children, and this is what I did. Many people ask me if I miss nursing, and most days the answer is no. But there are a few bright moments in my almost twenty years' experience that are fun to look back on. I miss the nurses I worked with, and toward the end of my career I missed the elderly patients the most.

I would sure like to read the journal of that nurse from the first hospital in Harrodsburg. No doubt she must have been a great and courageous woman.

According to Florence Nightingale,

> No man, not even a doctor, ever gives any other definition of what a nurse should be than this—"devoted and obedient." This definition would do just as well for a porter. It might even do for a horse. Nursing is an art, and if it is to be made an art, requires as exclusive a devotion, as hard a preparation, as any painter's or sculptor's work; for what is the having to do with dead canvas or dead marble, compared with having to do with the living body—the temple of God's spirit? It is one of the fine arts; I had almost said, the finest of fine arts.

Nightingale's words were obtained from her book *Notes on Nursing: What It Is and Is Not* (London: Churchill Livingston, 1859).

Bobbi Dawn Rightmyer, Harrodsburg, May 11, 2012

MEMORIES ABOUT MARY BRECKINRIDGE

I remember learning that Mrs. Breckinridge had fallen and broken her back a few years earlier than when I first met her. I can't remember too much about her appearance, but she was short, gray, and elderly. She had short hair with a fringe, or "bangs," as you call it. I don't think she was ever called Mary and was just called Mrs. Breckinridge. She never talked about things such as her husband and children, but she was from a fine old family from the South in America. I think her father was an ambassador, or maybe vice president, or something. Anyway, Mrs. Breckinridge was in the [social?] circle. . . .

Relative to her feelings about mountain people, she was always protective. I think she wanted to do as much as she could for 'em.

It is said that her reaction to black people was that she wouldn't sleep under the same roof with one of them. . . .

Mrs. Breckinridge usually kept a distance between herself and the staff, but she was always friendly to me. We were occupants of her house in Wendover and were conscious that it was her home and her house. We just worked there. She had lots of visitors from all over the world and entertained them. People used to come from all over the world to see how she and her work functioned. . . . She knew what was going on at every clinic.

She went out and gave speeches and raised money that way, and I had heard that even before I went over to Wendover.

Told by Lydia Thompson to Carol Crowe-Carraco, 1978;
provided by the Louie B. Nunn Center for Oral History,
University of Kentucky Libraries, Lexington

WORKING WITH NURSE-MIDWIVES IN INDIA

When I was in India we had our own nursing school and our own nurse-midwifery school, and the midwives did all normal deliveries of babies, and they had a lot. We were upward of two thousand deliveries a year, and the midwives did all but the abnormal ones. So I was accustomed to teaching midwives, working with midwives, and I do like the system.

The system was better staffed in India than in the FNS, but I had more to work with, had good equipment, thus was better equipped all the way around. And I called more of the signals myself as far as working personally. I got what I wanted and asked for.

Told by Dr. Mary Wiss to Dale Deaton, February 14, 1979;
provided by the Louie B. Nunn Center for Oral History,
University of Kentucky Libraries, Lexington

MIDWIVES' CONTINUATION SERVICES

I frankly think the midwife concept is excellent, both for the delivery of obstetrical care and the humaneness. I think the midwives should be working under a doctor's supervision and when there is a problem the doctor is immediately available. However, even with a complicated delivery I would support a midwife through it. I think most obstetricians would be better off, especially the really busy ones, to have a nurse-midwife or two in their offices for routine prenatal care and postpartum care and to sit down and talk with women who need somebody to talk to and to discuss their pregnancies and problems with. I think midwives have a great deal to offer.

Such a practice would be accepted by the patients in rural areas, but not by the doctors, who feel that their little nest is being invaded. I had a friend who was a practicing midwife in Frankfort, and because she doesn't practice it now is because there were doctors . . . obstetricians who just got a third partner in and he decided they were paying her too much money, that it was better off in their pocket. However, the patients followed her. . . . One of her patients was Governor Carroll's wife.

Told by Dr. Mary Wiss to Dale Deaton, February 14, 1979;
provided by the Louie B. Nunn Center for Oral History,
University of Kentucky Libraries, Lexington

NURSE'S MOVE FROM MICHIGAN TO KENTUCKY

I guess I first found out about the Frontier Nursing Service through the director of nurses at Harper Hospital in Birmingham, Michigan, back in the 1940s. I graduated from Harper in 1946. I was on staff at Harper after I finished school and was on staff until June 1947. I personally worked strictly in the clinic the whole time I was there at the hospital in Birmingham.

Two of us went down to the FNS in September 1947. Other than myself, the other nurse that went with me was Betty Scott, who has since passed away. At Frontier Nursing Service I worked as a clinic nurse in what is now the old hospital, and I was on duty every day in the clinic when it was open. I was also on call sometimes in the evenings when they brought in emergency cases such as shootings! There were probably more shootings cases back then than there are now because there were some family feuds going on in the area, or in the outlying area.

I went down to the FNS when I was told they wanted some nurses and that there was a midwifery school there too. I had to leave there in June 1948 because of family illness back up here in Michigan. To get to Hyden I went from Detroit to Lexington by train and from there to Hyden I rode a bus. In terms of what Hyden looked like when I got there in 1947, there were a lot of wooden buildings. There weren't too many buildings in Hyden other than the stores. The FNS provided me with living quarters upstairs at the hospital. The hospital had good facilities but they were not as modern as a city hospital. The hospital did have an operating room and a delivery room, plus the crib section for the newborns, and it also had a small x-ray room and two large rooms for the clinic.

Soon after I got there I met Mrs. Breckinridge. Sometimes on our day off we'd go over to Wendover, maybe to visit other nurse friends over there. We always tried to be there at teatime. At that time she was still active and would come to the hospital and go out to some of the centers close by. As to how she looked, she was short and was a very friendly looking person. She wore her hair very short and it was fairly gray. I seem to remember she always had a smile on her face, but occasionally when the conversation became serious or if she was upset about something the smile might disappear, but she was always a very friendly person with her staff.

As staff members we didn't have much opportunity [to socialize], but on our day off we were always together and sometimes we'd go out and visit some of our other nurse friends that were out in the centers or something like that. However, back in the 1940s our lives were pretty much centered around the Frontier Nursing Service even when you were off duty. Your life was centered around that because there wasn't an easy way to get anyplace else, but there were still a lot of horses being used for transportation and there were also a few jeeps.

Dr. Burney was the medical director when I got there, and Dr. Francis Nelson was at the surgical clinic. He and his two nurses had come to Hyden. And I think Betty Lester was at the hospital at that time and later on she went into social work.

Eva Gilbert was one of the ones in charge of School of Midwifery, and Doris "Red" Reed worked out of one of the small centers, too. She had red hair and we always called her "Red."

In reference to outpost clinics, Confluence was still a center when I was down there, and so was Bowlingtown, but both of them were closed when Buckhorn Dam was built in the area.

I don't remember what my salary was while I was in Hyden, but I do know it was much less than what I would have received elsewhere. However, I did get free room and board. My work at the FNS was an interesting type of work if you were willing to go off and be in an area where your time often was centered around your job. I didn't need a lot of pay because there wasn't a lot to do down there. [Laughter.]

I was an RN when I went down to Hyden, Kentucky. Let me say I had to assume more responsibility when I got there than I would have elsewhere. The gal that eventually left the clinic taught me how to do lab work on urinalyses and blood counts and those types of things. She also taught me how to run the x-ray machine, which wasn't a complicated one. It was very elementary. We did have a small pharmacy, and we filled prescriptions right there. All services required just minor charges if the patient could pay. Otherwise services were free. For patients that could pay, maybe twenty-five cents were charged for some medications, or a dollar for the x-ray or something like that.

Thinking back, let me say that in Hyden and surrounding areas it is a very pretty section of the country. Working there was more like serving grassroots people and in a way a lot more meaningful. Actually, I think it would mean even more today to the young nurses than it did to us. Young nurses of today don't have as much person-to-person contact with their patients as we used to have, and maybe they'd really enjoy the personal contact today down there. They certainly don't get it up here, I guess because so many of the registered nurses now have their bachelor's degree and they're either the head nurse or the medicine nurse or something like that rather than the individual taking care of patients or being familiar with patients.

Recently I was back in Hyden. It happened when my husband and I were down in Georgia, and coming up I-75 we got off and went down to see the new hospital, which is truly more modern and is beautiful.

Told by Nancy N. Porter to Dale Deaton, March 5, 1979;
provided by the Louie B. Nunn Center for Oral History,
University of Kentucky Libraries, Lexington

RATIONALE FOR COMING TO KENTUCKY

I took the two-year nursing course in Michigan, so I have an associate degree in nursing. I worked for about six months and then I went to Costa Rica and spent three years working there, which was very educational relative to a nursing job. While I was there I worked with Katie Yoder, who had taken her midwifery training here in Wendover, Leslie County. She suggested that I come here because I was a bit frustrated with what I was doing in Costa Rica, was not well prepared for it. Katie suggested that I come back to the United States and before considering another work term I should get more education.

She told me this would be a good place to work, especially in the midwifery program. I recall being impressed by the fact she was still writing letters to some of the local people here that she had taken care of when she was working here. What she wrote was so interesting to me, because she had been gone from here for four years before we had that interaction.

So I did work through the family nurse and midwifery programs here, and it took me sixteen months since I wanted to become both a family nurse practitioner and a midwife. By taking these courses individually, it would take twelve months to complete each one. Primarily

I think the FNS program gives you the skills of physical assessment. . . . I think a registered nurse is more on a one-to-one basis with the patient, whereas a family nurse is aware of the fact that husband affects the wife and maybe some of the wife's problems are due to their relationship.

We're very strong in counseling, not only about health care maintenance, and helping people to realize that they can do a lot for themselves in maintaining good health, thus preventing problems. Because we have these assessment skills we can set up baby clinics, doing annual physical exams, doing a lot of screening as far as adolescent clinics, clinics for women such as breast checks and pap smears. I always feel like now that I am a practitioner there is a certain part of my professional role that I can do independently of any physician, whereas a registered nurse is totally under the direction of a physician.

I've said a lot of things, but I think the basic difference between a registered nurse and family nurse is that we're more involved with the family unit, and we do have that portion that is independent of physicians.

Told by Karen Slabaugh to Dale Deaton, March 23, 1979;
provided by the Louie B. Nunn Center for Oral History,
University of Kentucky Libraries, Lexington

MEETING MARY BRECKINRIDGE
WAS A WONDERFUL EVENT

When I came down here to Wendover as an incoming student in 1962 I met Mary Breckinridge. What I initially knew about her was by reading through the history books relative to her reputation and what she had done here. I can't remember the first time I met her, but I think it was just at an informal tea [party]. We used to have tea at four o'clock every day at Wendover, and all the students got an opportunity to go over to meet Mrs. Breckinridge. At these get-togethers she was most relaxed and just welcomed us as a class to the school and to the FNS. I really didn't get into any formal discussion with her at the time. I was a shy girl when I first came to Wendover. All of the students respected her and were not fearful of her.

As a district nurse-midwife working at the Red Bird Center I got acquainted with Mrs. Breckinridge through the committee meetings we would have. At that time she was too elderly to come out to the centers; thus the annual meetings were held at Wendover. They had a special dinner, and a lot of the community members would come to Wendover and we'd have our annual meeting. So I began to know her a little bit better through that, and also just through working as a district nurse-midwife. I found her a very strong individual who was very much in control of everything within the Frontier Nursing Service and knew just about everything that was going on. Whether you told her or not, she found out!

I think the biggest thing was that she was very much concerned about war-patient care and that she wanted the very best quality of care given to the people, thus would do everything in her power to help us do that. So if there were certain rules that were perhaps formed to give some law and order to the running of the FNS, if there was a need for an exception because of a certain circumstance, she would always have a listening ear and would consider [the need] as an individual matter. And then she always had time for you. To do that you could make an appointment and come in to see her.

I guess one of my biggest impressions on my personal life from Mrs. Breckinridge has to do with when I planned on leaving FNS in 1964. I had planned on going back home and getting married, but about a week or so before I was to leave I had made a decision to change my mind about that. And so I went to see Mrs. Breckinridge and talked to her in the living room of the big house. I asked her if, indeed, I did make this decision not to marry would she consider having me come back on staff again? And I can still see her sitting on her chair and saying, "My dear, you always have a home here."

I think she ran the FNS as a family. Most of us were single women with families that were far away, but some had no families. Because of the latter she created a family atmosphere for us. She grouped us together at times, like Thanksgiving at Wendover or some of the other annual events. Any time that we wanted to come in and have dinner at Wendover, if we were busy district nurses and had to come into town, if we wanted to come into Wendover, we were always welcome. There was never a closed door, and you never had to make a reservation, as it was always available to you. Everybody worked hard, and she expected you to get your work done, but in the evening she wanted you to come in and relax and just share.

I've heard stories about back when she was younger that she would go out to the district centers and spend the evening with the district nurses. She didn't do that while I was here because she was already too old and sickly. Nevertheless, she welcomed us to come in to see her, and that's what made the difference, I think.

Told by Elsie Maier to Dale Deaton, December 5, 1978;
provided by the Louie B. Nunn Center for Oral History,
University of Kentucky Libraries, Lexington

EARLY MOUNTAIN WORKING YEARS

When I first came to this area I was at Beech Fork and the clinics there were held in the center several days each week. We had two nurses, two jeeps, and two horses, so we shared the work. . . . This is the way centers were set up back then; thus you were supposed to relieve each other until somebody went on vacation.

I took over when Ruth Vander Mullen left Beech Fork. She was going overseas, and she broke me in by taking me around the district on horseback to show me all the houses. While at Beech Fork my job was focused on the Stinnett area. We also had all the highway from Asher Post Office down to Stinnett and up the hill, because we had areas that were out of district, and that was the upper Muncy's Creek which was at the top of Stinnett Hill. And then I also had the downriver area towards Wendover, and there was no roadway there at all when I did it. You used to have to go down to the big river when it was low enough in order to drive your jeep right smack down into the middle of the river. It went down so far until it hit the road, and the road went down to Tug Point. We went down that road a little way, then had to take a boat to get over to the people on the other side. All of that took place in December 1955.

Back then all of the nurses lived in the centers and they were all midwives. . . .

Our great emphasis was on home visiting, and all the creek clinics were only to help people who couldn't get all the way out into the town of Hyden, or into us at Beech Fork, nor the nursing center. They were mostly medical clinics, but a great number of them were extra clinics such as worming clinics, which you set up. These clinics weren't always the same kind, but there was one steady prenatal clinic that was part of a wide area near Stinnett but it was called Grassy. Actually, it was always held in the living room at a Smith's house. The patients came around and sat and waited for service.

We rode every day on horseback because it was quicker to go on horseback and over the hill than it was to drive around up Stinnett and out into Grassy. So that was a permanent thing, a week clinic. Some of them were on Tuesday, and we went every day, even if it didn't matter how cold it was. I was there during a very cold winter and the temperature was at minus ten; thus it was quite cold in the house.

Told by Molly Lee to Eliza Culp, February 6, 1979;
provided by the Louie B. Nunn Center for Oral History,
University of Kentucky Libraries, Lexington

EARLY SERVICE YEARS

When I came here we did general nursing, thus just about anything that came around. We served both as district nurses and midwives. That was one of the reasons why I had a fair amount to offer, because I came to nurse's training because a district nurse's training prepared us to make do without in the homes, to do dressings, to use a cot or a little basin in which to put your solutions.

We were encouraged to be able to drop in and visit people as you were passing by, and you tried to organize your day so that you went in the same direction, to see people in that direction. So we were not going in a hundred different ways in one day.

If we were on horseback we saw people when we were passing by much more readily than if we were traveling in a jeep. One of the things that was so difficult as we passed by people is because where they lived was like a matriarchal society. It seemed to be that the mother and the grandmother of the family had an awfully strong say in things. I don't know why it was that way except that the men probably kept out of the medical part of it. If there were a baby delivery, the men were hardly ever around.

On one occasion we'd been left alone in a home in which the woman's husband had just left. Usually there were a lot of children when there was a home delivery taking place, so the men would sometimes take the children to a neighbor, or to another room. That's one of the reasons why men didn't hang out for the delivery.

Told by Molly Lee to Eliza Culp, February 6, 1979;
provided by the Louie B. Nunn Center for Oral History,
University of Kentucky Libraries, Lexington

AN EARLY NURSE IN HYDEN

During the fall, 1938, I went to the Bull Creek District and was there about eighteen months, then went to Flat Creek for about a year, then came to Hyden in 1940. The medical director we had then was Dr. Cooper, who asked me if I could come in and be hospital midwife. I'd had some difficult cases out at Flat Creek, which, according to him, I had handled very satisfactorily. I went in and it was hard work because I came in at the end of the year 1940. Within a year America went to war and we lost a lot of nurses, so I was in charge of the whole patient floor. I was sort of counselor for the nurses we had on the general side during the day. There was always a registered nurse on duty at night. I was working with volunteers on both sides. A lot of them were aides and we could never run the hospital without couriers. . . .

I would go over there in the morning and just give them the initial orders, such as which patients they were to give baths to, and if there were any very sick [patients] to go and look at them and say, "I'll come back later but I've got to do my duties to mothers and babies first."

Told by Helen E. Browne to Carol Crowe-Carraco, March 26, 1979;
provided by the Louie B. Nunn Center for Oral History,
University of Kentucky Libraries, Lexington

NURSES' SLOW LEARNING

After a few years as a nurse you get the job of mentoring new nurses, who are just as green if not greener than you were when starting out. After report, two of my newer nurses had the floor to themselves with sixteen patients, eight for each one. One older gentleman had "a bad ticker," as he called it, and back then no one was allowed to stay with a patient unless it was a special circumstance. This man had complained of intermittent chest pain on and off all day. Of course, I worked doubles when I could since good money could be made this way.

Nitro worked well every time for his chest pain, but Maalox and Tums also worked almost as well. The "almost" is what my nurses did not catch. Anyway, the night progressed and so did his discomfort. All of the important and necessary tests were completed and the physician notified at the appropriate intervals. All of a sudden the overhead paging system comes alive with the dreaded words, "CODE 500 room 205! CODE 500 room 205!" As we ran down the halls and into the room, there the patient was on the floor, completely unresponsive. One of the nurses looked up at me helplessly and said, "All I did was take him to the bathroom," whereas the other nurse responded, "That's what happened to Elvis!"

I was taken back by the frantic looks on their faces, both working hard to get the poor patient on his side. One nurse yelled out to the other nurse, "NOW shove the backboard under so I can get chest compression started." At this point I have to jump in and say, "Wait a minute, both of you; he is on the FLOOR and does not need a BACKBOARD under him for compression."

Needless to say, the gentleman lived at least long enough to get away from the new nurses who did not think the floor was hard enough, but it took a long time for them to live that one down.

In small hospitals word travels fast and stays longer.

Jana Buckles, Lawrenceburg, June 9, 2012

Early Nursing Career

Back when I came to Hyden in 1939 I was in the outpatient department, and we had one nurse part-time and one part-time clerk-steno, but we got the second nurse. Back then we generally averaged seventy-five to one hundred patients each day. We were very busy all the time, as we were also responsible for all emergencies. Clinic patients arrived anywhere from five in the morning through the rest of the day, and while officially we did not go to work until 8:00 a.m., usually by eight you had maybe ten or fifteen patients already seen. And when we had the second nurse, the two of us worked very well together.

The second nurse was Gladys Moberg, now Gay. We went to midwifery class together. We would prepare the patients that were to be seen by the nurse and take care of them, and the other prepared the patients and did all of the things that needed to be done before the doctors saw them. For example, if the patient had an infected lesion on the leg, and we used to have a lot of them, we went ahead and did the soaking, cleaning up, and prepared the patient for the physician to see them.

The physician then made rounds through those that he could see right on the spot and then left directions for the nurse to do it. And you went ahead and processed these according to the orders the doctor had wrote down on their cards. The ones that we had to see were prepared in the clinic office room. If it were a female patient, we prepared them in the clinic office room and then went in with them to see the doctor. There were instructions for birth control, for instance, and pelvic examinations. The nurse[s] assisted the doctor with all these things, or were at least present.

Told by Grace Reeder to Carol Crowe-Carraco, January 25, 1979;
provided by the Louie B. Nunn Center for Oral History,
University of Kentucky Libraries, Lexington

FROM ALBERTA TO HYDEN

The reason I came to Frontier Nursing Service took place when I was a student at Calby General Hospital in Alberta, Canada, and we would look through the nursing journals at the employment opportunities section and write letters because we were all broke little student nurses. We got paid only fifteen dollars each month, which was supposed to buy our stockings and our shoes. The Frontier Nursing Service had an ad in the *American Journal of Nursing*, and it said something about experience in rural nursing, isolation, and nurses on horseback. Well, I answered a number of ads in that publication, two of which were good enough to send me a reply; one was in Alaska and the other was the Frontier Nursing Service in Kentucky.

I have a little bit of the pioneer sense of adventure, but most particularly I had spent three years in a big hospital school in a good-sized city. I was raised on a ranch in the country, and I wanted the dirt of the city off my feet immediately. I had always thought about being a nurse in a rural area, and certainly what I learned about the Frontier Nursing Service sounded like the right place. The idea of good-looking horses didn't hurt anything. I grew up on a horse on the ranch.

I went to Hyden in the fall, 1958, and worked on the so-called general side of the Hyden Hospital. We didn't have a doctor at the time. We still had people in the hospital, and we were looking after them, so I got some experience real quick. I also learned to speak Kentuckian as opposed to Albertan, which helped.

On my way here I rode a Greyhound bus from Calgary in Alberta to Salt Lake City and then came east to Lexington. Seatbelts and staying in your seat were not heard of in that day, so I stood up alongside the driver and took pictures through the window most of the way. It was a long trip but I enjoyed it more or less, and when I got to Kentucky it was the day before Halloween. At Halloween in Alberta people dress up in silly costumes and run around begging treats at doors. Sometimes they even take Jack-o-lanterns and put them on the doorsteps of an old person and bang on the door and run. What I didn't know is that in eastern Kentucky people set fires, shoot guns, cut down trees in the road, do other weird stuff, so I thought, "What in the heck?"

Told by Jean Fee to Rebecca Adkins Fletcher, June 15, 2002; provided by the Louie B. Nunn Center for Oral History, University of Kentucky Libraries, Lexington

AN ACCIDENT AND SHOOTING

I remember being called to an accident where a car had fallen on a guy who was a mechanic, but he was under his car and had it rigged someway, but it became unrigged and the car fell on him. Some boys thereabouts had gotten the car off him but he was fairly well squashed. And while they sent for an ambulance, which was within range at that point, they had me to come and see about him and give him something for pain and make sure he was breathing all right, which he was.

I think that was the worst accident I got in on, but there were other stories at Wolf Creek before I came there. Somebody who reputedly was stealing timber was shot while on a bulldozer at the top of a mountain, but it was probably not the operator of the dozer that was in contention. But he was the guy that got shot, and from there a nurse was taken to the top of the mountain to see about the patient, which she did, and then the nurse and the patient both rode the bulldozer to the bottom of the mountain, and when the patient reached the hospital he recovered. To me, that was very dramatic.

Told by Jean Fee to Rebecca Adkins Fletcher, June 15, 2002; provided by the Louie B. Nunn Center for Oral History, University of Kentucky Libraries, Lexington

ARRIVAL ON THE MOUNTAIN

If you want to know the story as to why and how I came here to the mountains, I still wonder about it. I grew up in Canada and had my nurse training there. When I was in nursing school they asked me, "What are you going to do when you graduate?" I said, "I'm going to the Kentucky mountains to take care of the hillbillies."

That was my answer, but I'm not sure whether I really thought it or not. I had never read anything specific about the hillbillies, but had read some things that were intriguing, especially the language. As a child I had lived in a rural Texas area where I was born, in the Wild West. Then my parents moved back to Canada in a rural area when I was six years old. We had rural nurses there that did community work. That was my first contact with nurses that went from home to home. One of them came to our house one time when I was sick. I also know that she went to other places when they had babies. She didn't do health care, so I think that's what intrigued me about nursing and why I wanted to go into nursing. And, of course, our doctor was thirteen miles away. You never called a doctor unless you really needed one, which was not very often.

We weren't poor there in Canada like some of these people here in the mountains, but we didn't have roads. During the winter we were snowed in from November to May. We had horses and traveled by horseback. When it rained we rode horseback to school, or rode by carriage, but never by a car. So I was used to horses and loved them.

After I graduated from nursing I came back south right after that. The north was rather rugged. I had rheumatic fever, had a congenital heart, so they told me I should go to where it is warmer and more conducive to somebody who didn't have all the strength needed. So I worked in a small community hospital in Kansas where you were very closely tied with the community. It was thirteen miles from the nearest town, actually a little village. I learned a great deal there, thus really enjoyed my first year there. I soon had a patient there who was a sixty-year-old man and he was in the hospital all the time I was there.

That hospital was across the road from an old folks' home, and whenever residents needed skilled nursing care they were put in the hospital, and there were some that just stayed there. The hospital had only fourteen beds, and I had been there about nine months when one day this old fellow gave me a book. He was an old minister who was paraplegic at the time. He talked with great difficulty, but he was a delightful old gentleman anyway. When he gave me the book, he said, "This is where you belong."

One month later I was here in Kentucky, and I loved it during the minute I got here. I wanted to get into midwifery, but I wanted to work here awhile before I became a midwife. The hospital had a very hard time during World War II getting enough nurses, and they were just beginning to come back. I read an advertisement in a nurses' journal and was absolutely intrigued, so I answered it right off. Nurses were given responsibility from the minute you came here.

I spent about two weeks working in the hospital and then moved to Wendover.

Told by Gertrude Isaacs to Dale Deaton, November 15, 1978;
provided by the Louie B. Nunn Center for Oral History,
University of Kentucky Libraries, Lexington

Attendance at Nurse and Midwife Schools

I attended New England Baptist Hospital School of Nursing. I specialized about one and one-half months and then went right down to Kentucky to work in what we called the general side of the hospital in Hyden. I then decided that I wanted to do the midwifery course. So I worked at least six months and then went into a midwifery program on the scholarship basis, agreeing to stay for a year and one-half afterwards. I ended up staying almost eight and one-half years all total. Before I went to Kentucky I had no idea what floods were that ruined the land. We had a flood within two months after I got there. . . . I had a good idea of what the people were like. I read part of a book called *Wide Neighborhoods* before I got there and read the rest of it after I got there. I think I had a pretty good idea what the people were like, but until I experienced it I don't think I had really felt it inside. But I always liked the country after I got there, loved horses, and loved the people, [who were] not necessarily rich, plus I was very idealistic and wanted to cure the world.

Midwifery training at that time took up six months, so I worked like six months in the general hospital, getting to know the area, and then the midwifery course took six months. After that I worked on a scholarship basis for eighteen months as a midwife, not as a student.

Some of the nurses that went down there had a public health background. The first six months I was there I went with public health nurses on a lot of my days off, and I picked up a lot of information. What I learned was not necessarily taught as a prime in the midwifery courses, but I think a lot of it was intermingled with our courses. During that time Wendover set up the record system so we really had a good way to do things. We could adapt whatever we wanted to. Later on I became the only midwife there and worked jointly with an excellent public health nurse, Carolyn Coleman, who is now in Chicago.

Told by Mary Penton to Dale Deaton, June 15, 1979;
provided by the Louie B. Nunn Center for Oral History,
University of Kentucky Libraries, Lexington

QUEEN'S NURSE MEMORIES

I'm Molly Lee and I'm from Plymouth, Devon, England, and my general training was in England during the war, and then I did midwifery training in two places in Scotland, which were Stirling and Aberdeen. And then I did Queen's Nurses training in Exeter, Devon, England, which is a six-months' district nurses training, teaching us to do without, which is probably my greatest pleasure in life. After that I did three and one-half years on district in a rural area that had several small villages. I looked after everybody from virtually the cradle to the grave. I birthed them and buried them.

Then I got interested in the Frontier Nursing Service through Mary Green in Devon, to whom I was sent for a day's experience as a Queen's Nurse trainee. I decided that Kentucky was too populated and too civilized, so I went to Canada in 1952 for nearly three years in the Red Cross Outpost Service.

Let me say it was an honor to be a Queen's Nurse. Mrs. Breckinridge in Leslie County was very proud in having Queen's Nurses. I think that was because they were midwives and could take care of a whole scope of medical care in the home according to a doctor. They took care of medical things, surgical things, pediatric, and delivered babies at home. Care of the old people and teaching in the homes was really a big everything.

I rode a bicycle during the early days of training [in Canada], but we had a car in the villages because we couldn't cover the distance any other way. When I drove a car for the Queen's Nurses was the first time I ever had a car. But when I found out about horses being used for riding purposes I became interested in the horseback idea. It was a kind of utopia to have a horse and a dog and work all at the same time, which is what I found later. There just wasn't enough work to keep me in Canada after nearly three years. However, while I was there we had a lot of Indian patients who were members of the British Columbia Province. Not many of them were white, but I did their baby deliveries. I sometimes gave up my own bed and delivered the babies in my bed. It was only a three-bed outpost and we sometimes had as many as nine people there, counting the babies. So I stayed up at night with them and looked after the new babies until I got beyond it at times. The mothers had to take over then. On the other hand, we weren't always busy, but we took everything besides deliveries, including sick [adult] patients as well.

Told by Molly Lee to Carol Crowe-Carraco, February 6, 1979;
provided by the Louie B. Nunn Center for Oral History,
University of Kentucky Libraries, Lexington

Baby's Burial

After I arrived at Wendover around 1938 I remember two of us going from one center to the other. Almost always the two couriers went together, but I remember on one occasion when I went by myself to Red Bird. When I got there I saw this group of people standing and/or carrying this little box and so I stopped and talked to them. They were on their way to bury this baby. So I put the little casket in front of me and we went up to the cemetery. The baby's parents and several other children walked along beside me.

There weren't many deaths back then.

Told by Martha Webster, Appletree, OH, to Dale Deaton, March 4, 1979; provided by the Louie B. Nunn Center for Oral History, University of Kentucky Libraries, Lexington

Caring for Cows and Horses

Couriers had to care for the horses at Wendover. I also remember that every outpost center had to have a cow. So one day Marion Shouse and I had to take a cow from Wendover to Red Bird, or Beech Fork. I'm not sure which it was. Well, believe me, if you ever had to lead or drive one cow a considerable distance, whew!

I seem to remember going there because of a sick horse and Jean Hollands asked me to stay and help take care of it. I remember getting a big kick out of that, and I also remember how much admiration I had for all these mountain people. I also remember that Kermit Morgan helped take care of the horses [that were needed on an everyday basis].

Told by Martha Webster, Appletree, OH, to Dale Deaton, March 4, 1979; provided by the Louie B. Nunn Center for Oral History, University of Kentucky Libraries, Lexington

Primary Years Working for the FNS

During the summer of 1963 or '65, while I was in nursing school at Berea College, I applied for a courier job with the Frontier Nursing Service and was accepted. I wound up working mostly as a nurse's aide in the hospital in Hyden, Leslie County. I worked there and also worked in a couple of outpost centers. I wasn't paid to work as a courier. It was a volunteer job and was a really good experience, which I truly enjoyed.

Told by Martha Hill, Glendale, to Mark Brown, June 30, 2012;
provided by the Kentucky Historical Society, Frankfort

MARY BRECKINRIDGE'S FUNERAL

I read a lot of books about nursing before beginning my nursing education at Berea College. In the summer of 1964, before beginning my junior year at Berea, I applied for and was accepted for the job as courier at the Frontier Nursing Service. All the couriers had the opportunity at varying time[s] during their stay to visit the headquarters of the FNS at Wendover. During their visit they had the pleasure of meeting Mary Breckinridge, founder of FNS.

I'm not sure just when I went over to Wendover, but I think it was by invitation. When I got there, Betty Lester, who was in charge of the buildings, grounds, and the care of horses, took me up to the big house and introduced me to Mary Breckinridge. I also met Helen Browne (Brownie), who was the assistant director. Brownie became the director of FNS after Ms. Breckinridge died.

I remember having tea with Mary Breckinridge and talking for a while. She asked me where I was going to nursing school. I told her Berea College but I don't remember a response. I learned several years later that FNS and Berea College had some connections. Kate Ireland, who was resident courier in the early years of FNS, later served on the Board of Trustees of Berea College. Ms. Breckinridge also asked me what I was going to do after graduation. I don't remember my response, but at one time I thought about becoming a midwife.

Mary Breckinridge died in 1965, during my senior year at Berea College. I had the opportunity to go with President Dr. Frances S. Hutchins and his wife to the funeral. I appreciated that opportunity, and I guess I must have said something to Dr. Louise Hutchins, wife of the president, about having worked there at FNS in Leslie County.

Mrs. Breckinridge was very well known for her work in eastern Kentucky and the founding of the Frontier Nursing Service and the Frontier Graduate School of Nurse Midwifery and Family Nursing. I can't remember for certain, but I think her funeral was conducted in Frankfort and there was a large number of people there.

Told by Martha Hill, Glendale, to Mark Brown, June 30, 2012;
provided by the Kentucky Historical Society, Frankfort

Pleasant Career Memories

When we were going through our rotation in surgery, we had to put on a sterile gown and sterile gloves, and for some reason there wasn't a lot of extra equipment (tables) in the room to use to spread the pack out and get the gown and gloves on. There was this little stool that you turned around and around to increase the height or whatever. Our sterile packet was on that stool, so we had to make sure that we were standing a suitable short distance [away] and were careful so that we wouldn't knock it off onto the floor.

Another thing I remember as a student is about an instructor whom I really liked a lot. We got to the point of learning how to start intravenous fluids and had to choose a partner to give and receive an IV stick. As luck would have it, I had an instructor as my partner and I had to stick her. This was rather intimidating, but I managed to get it in the very first time and was very proud of myself.

Told by Martha Hill, Glendale, to Mark Brown, June 30, 2012;
provided by the Kentucky Historical Society, Frankfort

Successful and Nonsuccessful Students

I had one lady in nursing school whom I don't remember whether or not she finished the program. She was just too nervous around patients to become a really good nurse.

I had another student who was very smart but was also very nervous around patients, so I told her, "You know, I think it would be good for you to work in a research type of hospital where you'd have to do a lot of detailed things but hands-on contact with patients would be minimal."

I think she went to Vanderbilt Hospital in Nashville to work in the research unit, and I assume she had a successful career.

Most of our students that went through our Elizabethtown Community College were very successful in doing hands-on work with patients because we emphasized clinical skills and had as many clinical hours in the program that we could. There was one lady who was a straight-A student, but she had difficulty applying things in the clinical area. I don't think she successfully passed the clinical evaluation, thus likely failed her last nursing class. We had lots of students who failed before they even got to the last course. Many came back, repeated the course, and were successful. We had very few students who failed their state board exam and did not practice nursing. Only three or four did during the thirty years I was at the college.

Our program was really a strong program, and I think our students were very successful when they completed school and became nurses.

Typically I did not see many of the students after graduation, but many went on to earn higher degrees in nursing, even a Ph.D.

Told by Martha Hill, Glendale, to Mark Brown, June 30, 2012;
provided by the Kentucky Historical Society, Frankfort

STRESSED TEACHER'S CORRECT DECISION

One time we had a student [in nursing school] who failed, so he went to see the president and complained about failing. The president called in three of us instructors who taught in that class and asked for an explanation.

It was sort of a stressful time, and I said to him, "Do you think we didn't grade fairly? In our opinion we feel that we did, so maybe there's nothing else to talk about."

I got up and started to leave and the president banged his fist on the desk and said, "Sit down, young lady, I'm not finished talking with you yet."

That was sort of stressful, but he did not ask us to change the grade. We worked out a compromise; we would give the student another chance to take a final exam, and if he passed it we would change his grade and pass him. So we told the student and then set a date to give him enough time to study more if he needed to. Well, he did not pass that exam either, so he had to come back and repeat the course.

The president never said any more about it. Years later he said something to me referring to that event; he said that I was the only coordinator for that program who was not afraid to stick her neck out for her beliefs.

I said, "Thank you; that was the only way I could operate back then. I had to stand up for my beliefs and hang on to them if I thought I was right."

So he complimented me on that characteristic and we got along famously after that.

Told by Martha Hill, Glendale, to Mark Brown, June 30, 2012;
provided by the Kentucky Historical Society, Frankfort

MEMORIES OF YESTERDAY

One time we went back to Berea College for a homecoming and I was talking to the chairman of the music department because I had always been interested in music. He and I were walking together along the sidewalk and my husband, Danny, was walking behind us with one of my former nursing faculty members when I was a student. I said to the chairman that some people must have thought I was a music major because I liked music when I was in college and I was music director of our church choir and was also singing in a gospel quartet.

My nursing instructor, walking along behind us, said, "Well, Martha, there were times when I thought that, but you have since ex-onerated yourself."

She knew I was very active and worried about me at one time as to whether or not I was to be a nurse. However, according to her I clari-fied that and had gotten on track. Her name was Martha Pride, and she was one of my favorite nursing instructors. However, she taught the psychiatric course in nursing that I liked least of all the courses. I could never have been a psychiatric nurse. She was really a favorite teacher for a lot of students at Berea. She passed away this past year, but just before her passing four of the 1966 class got to visit with her at our forty-fifth class reunion.

Told by Martha Hill, Glendale, to Mark Brown, June 30, 2012;
provided by the Kentucky Historical Society, Frankfort

NURSING SERVICE ACROSS THE YEARS

During my early years of direct patient care I observed nurses in worse physical condition than the patients for whom they were providing services. There was no retirement for nurses other than the ones who worked in governmental health care entities such as veterans hospitals, public health, miners hospitals, etc. I had hoped to make it better for nurses, so I tried and think I did, even if for a very few.

As previous years passed the demands for nurses changed and the entire profession changed. It seemed in the rising of nursing to a more professional status, the nurse became less professional. It certainly has been true in appearance. I had to end the direct patient-care positions because the staff-patient ratio increased and the level of care required for the acute-care patient was so intense that I could not go home at night without worrying about all the patients I was able to care for. I am thankful I lived during the time of so much progress in technology and was able to master it all.

There are some images of unusual or amusing experiences which have left permanent pictures on the canvas of my brain, thus on my life as well.

The following poem about "Porter and Maggie" was written by me and published in my book *Patterns of Grace: The Poetry of Aging:*

Come meet two of my former patients,
A nursing home room they did share
Maggie was blind; Porter became her eyes
Finding, picking up, helping her

He was kind. Her mind had slipped, or had it?
"Porter, I lost my comb," she said to mate
Frail as he was under the bed he went
Crawling for Maggie, deliberate

Day in and day out he would meet her needs;
She contrived to keep him near her hand
Porter this and Porter that it did seem
Though they each understood the commands

The nurses would come to help as needed,
Then one morning when a still
Penetrated the room reverently
Quietly sitting slumped by her bed

No answer, no movement, just sitting there,
Porter dressed for his daily tasks
He had fallen asleep when breathing ceased
He had given all that was asked

"Porter, Porter, help me," was softly heard
"Porter, Porter, please answer me,
Porter, Porter, where are you?" she asked again
"Porter's gone. He loved you Maggie."

Evelyn Pearl Anderson, London, July 18, 2012

NURSE SERVICE TIME IN MAYSVILLE

My nursing career began in September 1961 with my first position as a staff nurse at Hayswood Hospital in Maysville, Kentucky. It was there we had to work thirteen consecutive days in order to get a long weekend off. Sometimes you wondered if a long weekend was worth it. A long weekend consisted of Friday, Saturday, Sunday, and Monday. After that it was back to work. My salary was great! I seem to remember I made ninety cents per hour. It cost twenty dollars a month to live in the nurses' residence. It had a kitchen and a nicely furnished lobby, used to entertain guests. Nurses had their meals furnished in the hospital's cafeteria. It was easy to get credit downtown at the Merz's Department Store because everyone in town knew that nurses had "good salaries."

It was a big step to leave the hospital where one had been schooled and where most of one's friends were living. However, it seemed right to go to Maysville, where the only hospital was located, near Flemingsburg, my home of origin. Even though it was near home, I really didn't know anyone. It seems transition was shaping up to remain my entire life. I was a new nurse and another new nurse was Madeline, with whom I became a good friend. I had another friend in town by the name of Patti, who had just graduated from a college in Ohio. She taught special education at the local school. Patti and I had known each other for a number of years. It was a busy time and the work was so demanding that there was little time for social life activities; thus there was very little energy left for keeping up with old friends.

Nursing was exciting back then since it was before specialties grew up in health-related problems. There would be persons on the same floor being treated for heart attacks, fractured hips, pneumonia, and sometimes children and elderly people were on the same floor. This was not good for infection-control management, but it was wonderful for learning and building self-esteem with enthusiasm.

The nurse's uniform is very important. It signifies her rank in school, and the right to wear it has been earned by long hours of careful preparation. A neatly dressed nurse is a credit to her whole profession. A complete uniform is a beautiful thing. This is the way we were taught and this is what we believed. We would have been totally shocked at the scrub dress and tennis shoes of today['s] on-the-job look.

There was no air conditioning, so on hot days we would rush around doing the ordered and necessary treatments and giving the medications on schedule. We would be so hot that sweat would roll down the back of our legs, covered in our heavy white stockings. There was not such a thing as pantsuits at that time, and our caps were pinned neatly to our hair. We worked hard and perspired but never missed a beat and remained looking good in the process. Of course, those white clinic shoes were shining, just like we had been taught in nurses' school to keep [them].

Evelyn Pearl Anderson, London, July 18, 2012

IMPORTANCE OF NURSES BACK THEN

Back then it was the time when the physician was mighty important in the hospital. The nurses would stop any and all charting at the desk to stand at attention when the doctor would come. There were no heart monitors or intensive care units for patients with cardiac problems to be rushed off to. I learned that I could count a pulse as rapidly as the electrocardiogram strip could mechanically read the pulse.

We nurses would intervene and care for these patients as dictated by the physicians. The patient was in God's and our hands. We did what we could do and were usually successful. The physicians were good to leave their offices and come up on the hill when needed, but the nurse must be very sure the physician was needed. There were no wires to hook up and connect to an electronic outlet. There were no buttons to push except for the old elevator to get to the second floor.

Intravenous fluids were given at a slow drip. Tape was placed on the glass bottle of fluid to show the amount of fluid remaining at the end of a shift. Blood was rarely given, and when it was the physician would administer.

Evelyn Pearl Anderson, London, July 16, 2012

YOUNG DOCTOR WAS SMOKING

One day when I first began working at Hayswood Hospital a young man came walking down the hallway smoking a cigarette. Yes, people smoked in hospitals back then and for several years afterward. He was walking, seemingly nonchalant, toward the open area at the end of the hallway where the oxygen tanks were stored.

I called out to him, "Young man, young man, please put out your cigarette." He didn't seem to hear, so I repeated more forcefully, "Young man, put out your cigarette," and he then complied. Later that morning

I learned the "young man" was a new medical doctor. He had recently joined the hospital staff.

I felt embarrassed at my comments but knew it was a correct admonition, and he didn't seem to mind.

Evelyn Pearl Anderson, London, July 18, 2012

SUCCESSFUL EXAMINATIONS

I always loved dressing up in white to go to work. I was so proud to put on my white cap with a black stripe before beginning work. I was in love with my profession and my patients. I did not like working the 11:00–7:00 p.m. shift, six straight weeks of it.

Back then it was a time when you could get to know your patients, who stayed for several days.

One spring morning in 1962 a patient called me into her room to look out the window. Although I detest snakes, I have to admit what we watched was interesting. Little baby snakes had been born, but it was good that there was a wall and glass window between the snake and me.

I passed my registered nurse examination the second time around. It was okay that a graduate nurse could sign "graduate nurse" on the medical records until the strenuous examination was taken the second time. After that took place the curtains would close. It was truly a frightening time, and such a relief was found when the notice arrived to congratulate me for being a registered nurse in the state of Kentucky.

I believe my salary was increased to one dollar an hour.

Evelyn Pearl Anderson, London, July 18, 2012

YOUNG GIRL'S DEATH

Oneida is a small mountain village where the Oneida Baptist Institute and the Oneida Mountain Hospital were located. The village was about fifteen miles outside of Manchester, county seat of Clay County, Kentucky.

Nothing terribly eventful happened here related to direct patient care, other than finding an abnormality in an Oneida Baptist Institute student's urinalysis results. The student was a beautiful young girl from Michigan. A report was sent to her parents, who had follow-up examinations done.

The student died soon afterwards from a congenital kidney disorder. I suppose the abnormal laboratory report alerted the parents, who would otherwise have been shocked by their daughter's untimely death.

Evelyn Pearl Anderson, London, July 18, 2012

SANITARY HOSPITAL IN ONEIDA

While I was working in Oneida it was interesting to work with Dr. Chu, who had been a personal nurse for Chiang Kai-shek before attending medical school. Dr. Chu had been honored on Ralph Edwards's early television show *This Is Your Life*. He was a delightful gentleman in every sense of the word. And he was a very meticulous surgeon.

I remember how amazed I was to learn that there had been no postsurgical wound infections. I had been working in Louisville, where that had been a problem in the hospitals, but there in the mountains in Kentucky in that little hospital everything was as neat and clean as could be.

Evelyn Pearl Anderson, London, July 18, 2012

GREAT SERVICE IN ST. LOUIS, MISSOURI

My husband had enrolled in graduate school at Washington University, St. Louis, Missouri. He accepted a pastorate at the East Carondelet First Baptist Church in East Carondelet, Illinois, which was located across the Mississippi River from South County, St. Louis. We lived in a mobile home parsonage.

During the university's fall and spring semesters I worked the 11:00–7:00 p.m. shift at the university's health service. In between the semesters and summer I worked [the] 3:00–11:00 a.m. shift at the Centerville Township Hospital's intensive care unit. I did not function well on the seven-to-eleven shift, but this was the ideal time for me to work, with a husband in school and three children in kindergarten, first, and second grades. It was not a working situation that would maximize my skills as a registered nurse, but there were people who needed medical care. The patients were students at Washington University that would be admitted from the day clinic for influenza, nausea and vomiting, manic depressive disorders, or other conditions making the student too ill for the dormitory but not ill enough to be hospitalized. The infirmary also served as a late-night clinic for the university.

The primary challenge was to get the student patient in bed at an early hour so he/she would heal from their illness and be able to return to the classroom quickly. One student, Mary, was frequently admitted to the infirmary for depression. She would be so unable to express herself that she would stand for many minutes before saying anything, until her feet turned blue. She was very intelligent and was able somehow to keep her grades up. Mary was indeed a challenge, and I have often wondered if she graduated and if she were ever able to function on her own.

The more interesting students would come for services through the night clinic. One young woman came for medical help with a specific problem. She brought her huge dog with her, and he remained downstairs, lying on his owner's beautiful long black wool coat. The coat looked very expensive, even with the long white-gray fur from the dog over most of the coat. Somehow I could hardly believe that student patient when she said that she was a St. Louis grade-school teacher, as I wondered if she wore that coat to school for the little children to see.

That was an interesting employment there in St. Louis. The students seemed to always have something new to discuss with me, and the university provided Social Security, so that I never was concerned about my personal safety.

Evelyn Pearl Anderson, London, July 18, 2012

Working Part-Time at Historical Hospital

In 1973 we moved to Campbellsville in Taylor County, Kentucky. I had decided to not work outside the home for a while and was certain I would not tell anyone that I was a nurse. Our children were all in their early years of grade school, so I thought I needed to be at home, at least until they adjusted.

We moved into our house on Bell Avenue. Our telephone was quickly installed the next day. That very day, the phone rang. I answered, and the caller said, "Mrs. Anderson, this is the administrator at Jane Todd Crawford Memorial Hospital in Greensburg, Kentucky, and I have called to offer you a job."

I could hardly believe my ears, so I asked him how he knew I was a registered nurse. Of course, he had read it in the newspaper. Campbellsville College had published information about my husband joining their faculty, and they just happened to write that I was a registered nurse.

It seemed being a nurse was news that quickly traveled. I did eventually go there to work part-time.

Evelyn Pearl Anderson, London, July 18, 2012

A LONG, WINDING ROAD

I knew from an early age that I wanted to work somewhere in the medical field. My dream was to attend medical school at either University of Louisville or Duke University.

After completing high school at Hazel Green High School in Laurel County, I was accepted into Berea College and was very excited to be launching my career. That didn't last very long, as I soon met with my counselor to arrange the plan for me to meet my goal. I was very upset to hear that I had nowhere close to the curriculum on transcript that would make an easy path to medical school.

We did not have counselors in my high school during the late 1950s, so I had simply taken all the science courses I could find, believing I was preparing myself adequately. To my dismay, the counselor told me I would need to take at least two years of general college courses before taking any premed subjects. I will never forget the counselor saying, "Don't worry, if you work with me I will have you practicing medicine by the time you are twenty-seven or twenty-eight years old."

Twenty-seven or twenty-eight? I was seventeen, thus that was my lifetime away! So a crushed young seventeen-year-old who was already homesick dropped out. I returned to my hometown of London, Kentucky, and enrolled in Sue Bennett Junior College with history as my declared major. It lasted for one year.

In August of that same year the Berlin Wall was put up and President Kennedy made his plea to the nation, which included these words: "Mothers, prepare to say goodbye to your sons; wives prepare to say goodbye to your husband."

I felt obligated to sign up, so on October 17, 1961, I enlisted and signed up to be a medic. That didn't work either. Because of my test results I was convinced by a recruiting official that I should enlist in the intelligence service. Well, then I found myself enjoying military life, so I opted to pursue a career as an army officer. I served in Panama during the Cuban crisis of 1962, two full, one-year tour[s of] duty in Vietnam, with a two-year tour in Berlin, Germany, sandwiched in between.

After ten years of service, [with] the war in Vietnam winding down and, in turn, promotions slowing down, I decided to end my military service. I still had the urge to be somewhere in the medical field and decided to go back to school part-time in pursuit of my life's dream.

After working for a few years in order to save money for college and taking a few night courses at the same time, I entered the nursing program at George Mason University in Fairfax, Virginia, at the ripe ol' age of forty. I had mapped out a five-year plan to complete a four-year degree while working at least part-time. During that five years I pumped gas, worked as a night auditor at a motel, and interrupted my studies one summer and sold cars at a Nissan dealership across the Potomac in Maryland. Finally, right on schedule, at age forty-five I received my BS in nursing and realized my childhood ambition of working in the medical field.

For the next twenty-two years I worked in a field I dearly loved and believe that I contributed to the lives of each patient I was privileged to work with. Although I worked in cardiac ICU for about three years, my first love was always the emergency room. I worked in the third-busiest ER in the state of Virginia for over sixteen years before opting for the more lucrative job as an "agency," or contract, nurse.

I retired on my sixty-sixth birthday with absolutely no regrets about my career choice. If I could change anything, I would have gotten out of the army earlier and gone back to school much sooner than I did.

George W. Williams, London, September 21, 2012

Caring for Dying Patients

When I was a student nurse I worked at HMH and went to school during the week. I had already had experience with patients dying. As a student I will never forget we were given a critically ill patient. One of my classmates' patient[s] had died, and of course we had to clean him up. See, people didn't realize that when you die you defecate and urinate on yourself, so the girls were freaking out.

When they went to turn him he let out all the breath he had in his lungs, so one of the girls went screaming out the door and others refused to touch him. When his eyes opened a few more went running out of the room, and by this time I was laughing so hard that tears were rolling down my face. I explained to the remaining few that this was normal for when a person dies.

As we tagged his toe and were taking him to the morgue, of course we had to take an elevator, so [when] the patient sat straight up on the stretcher, and those girls had nowhere to go, so I thought they were all going to pass out. I just pushed him back down. It was so funny when they were trying to tell our instructor about it. You could see she was refraining from laughing her ass off!

Teresa Fryman Bell, Edmonson County, October 29, 2012

THE NURSE THAT ALMOST WASN'T

I grew up in a Christian home and I thought I had faith in the Lord to see me through.

However, that faith was tested all through nursing school until the end of training. As a matter of fact, that faith is still tested daily, and I would like to share a little of my life's testament.

First of all, the odds of my becoming a nurse were close to zero. I recall early in my life when asked that old question, "What do you want to be when you grow up?"

I reminisce saying that I would like to teach. At some point in my life I even said, "I would never want to be a nurse." Well, that old saying is right, "Never say never."

Here is where God had a plan for my life, as he does for everyone. Somehow, about midway through college, I changed my major from elementary education to nursing. Different people would just come up to me and say, "You would make a good nurse."

Nursing school was competitive in the process of getting into the program. I was lucky to get into the program on the first application attempt. Again, God has a plan. I remember crying [at] my first clinical when I couldn't make up a bed the way nurses were supposed to make a bed. Nursing students were checked off on everything. In my head I began thinking I was going to quit, but God led me further. Many cries later and long nights of not sleeping, I had somehow managed to graduate nursing school. I applied for a job with a local hospital and was hired easily. All of my references were good, and I had a good grade average. However, there was one more step needed that would make me an official RN. That step was passing the State Nursing Board's exam.

While I waited a few weeks for my exam results to come in the mail, I could work for the hospital as an RN applicant, meaning I still was not "official." During this time, there came several more cries and long nights of feeling overwhelmed, exhausted, and feeling as if I hadn't done enough for my patients. Don't get me wrong; most of the time I held my composure at work. However, upon arriving home the pressure would break like a water faucet turned on at full blast. God saw me through each night, as I prayed that his hands would guide my hands. After all, these patients were his patients to heal.

Finally, the weeks passed and the exam results were in the mail. I remember opening the letter while sitting in my car by myself. Here came the water faucet again. I had failed the test. Of course, what did I do except question God. Why did he want me to be a nurse, get me all this way, only to fail the test and be set back? Well, there was Satan trying to get in between God and me. I had to view it that way. I continued to work at the hospital as a nursing assistant until I could retake the exam. I did say to myself, "If I fail a second time. I will not try again." I firmly believe God has a plan for everyone, so guess what, I passed! Maybe God just thought I needed some extra time to adjust to work routine.

Not sure, but this is what prayer does. It is not answered the way one wants it answered, but it does get one through some mighty tough problems. Sometimes the hope of something is better, or the belief God will see you through regardless of the outcome is all one needs.

"Never say never" resurfaced again when I ended up becoming a staff nurse in the CCU/ICU [critical care unit/intensive care unit]. I started my career on a regular nursing medical floor, but after about three years I found myself in this specialty unit. Truthfully, I had said I didn't want to work there. This was the beginning of a long journey as a nurse. The journey was to be the best nurse I could be, with God on my side. Sticking with that was not easy. So many nights as I worked night shift I would think, "I can't do this anymore." Seeing pain, suffering, and death takes life out of a nurse's emotional well-being. But God continued to see me through. He was doing his work through me.

After twenty-two years as a nurse in a hospital, I did change jobs to work at a nursing school. Somehow I hoped to instill in students some of the experiences and/or learning I endured. Well, what was my first choice when I grew up? Does being a teacher ring a bell? As I write this, I'm still not teaching directly. My title is nursing lab coordinator. In other words, I just assist everyone else with all kinds of duties. Some days I do not feel important at all. To be a teacher means going back to school for at least a master's degree. Who knows where my life will take me? I've also heard, "You are never too old!" Well, I'm still talking to God about that one. Praying that I make the right choices, I must remember that his plan outweighs anything that I can come up with.

As I bring this account to an end, I feel it has this moral: If you truly want to be a nurse (or any other profession for that matter), just keep trying, hang in there, and let God lead the way. "Never say never" might just turn into "always say always."

Rebecca Collins, Auburn, January 31, 2013

CHANGES IN PAST FIFTY YEARS

When Joyce Parrish studied nursing at Louisville General Hospital, student nurses made $1.25 per hour.

She said, "We went to the University of Louisville that first year except for nursing classes at the hospital. During your junior you came and worked on the floor. It was free labor for the hospital. We had interns, residents, and student nurses."

Joyce was a Dunbar native and has seen changes since she began working at the Logan Memorial Hospital a little more than fifty years ago. She is currently a staff nurse who works in the hospital's operating room and recovery. She said, "We assess patients after surgery."

While she used to work more, she has cut back to working only two days a week. She said to me as she laughed, "There comes a time when you can't get on your knees and get up as easily. Initially I was going to enroll in Bethel College in Hopkinsville to be a teacher because the aunt who raised me was a teacher."

The rest of the story is that when a friend . . . told Parrish that she was going to Louisville for nurse training, Parrish also decided to go. It is of interest to note that back then the students were required to stay single. She went on to say, "Ours was the first class in which students were allowed to get married."

Her first job at Logan Memorial was as operating room supervisor. That was January 2, 1959. She was already familiar with the hospital because she had previously worked there as a nurse['s] aide. She said, "We were really busy since we were working supervisors and didn't have an office. We worked side-by-side with the rest of the staff doing bedside care and other work that supervisors often don't have to do now. We washed and sterilized gloves and syringes. We were M.A.S.H. in those days. We put linens up ourselves, and didn't have a lot of antibiotics except penicillin. Doctors also wore a variety of hats!

"We didn't have emergency room doctors there, but there were doctors who would come in for emergencies. Family doctors would give anesthesia. Family practice doctors did deliveries and took care of families."

Parrish remembers the mid-1960s when Medicare started. People wanted to make sure older people received as much care as possible. She said, "Medicare had a big effect on hospitals. We were full all the time."

Although Parrish has been working at Logan Memorial for a long time, she doesn't plan to retire immediately. In her words, "I enjoy my career, and I've made a lot of wonderful friends with patients and employees."

From Alyssa Harvey, "Logan Memorial Nurse Has Seen Much Change in Past 50 Years," Bowling Green Daily News, *July 24, 2010*

EARLY TRIP TO HINDMAN SETTLEMENT SCHOOL

I took a trip with Fay Smith at her request. The Kentucky school nurses needed their continuing education in domestic violence, and I had written with a social worker and a lawyer a program on domestic violence to fulfill that requirement for continuing education units.

So we were invited to speak to the Kentucky school nurses, and we presented the program and it went very well and was well received. Afterwards Fay asked me if I wanted to ride home with her, and I said, "Sure." So the other two went on back to northern Kentucky and I stayed with Fay as we traveled through some back roads in Kentucky to meet her Aunt Jack. So we met and visited with Aunt Jack. Fay then wanted to take me on to Hindman Settlement School in 1997. I had never been there. Believe it or not, while there I got to meet James Still, and that was quite an honor. I found him to be a very engaging gentleman, and I very much enjoyed visiting with him. I also was able to pick up a tape about Appalachian music from one of the young women who was also studying there.

That was a very interesting experience.

Patricia A. Slater, Petersburg, March 6, 2013

HUMOROUS BUT SERIOUS LIFE-SAVING EVENT

When I began my nursing career at Booth Hospital in 1965, CPR was just beginning to be taught to the staff. CPR training had not been a part of my nursing education in the Department of Nursing at Berea College.

Shortly after we were trained in CPR, a patient needed this life-saving skill. The day after we resuscitated her, she was sitting in her chair when her pastor came to visit. As I passed her room, I heard her minister ask, "How are you today?" In her shaky old lady voice, she responded, "Very well, but they broke my ribs saving my life yesterday."

The fact of the matter was that a rib had been broken during deep compressions. It appeared that she was not blaming the staff for breaking a rib as they worked to save her life.

Clara Fay Smith, Erlanger, March 6, 2013

ROACH VISITATIONS NOT FAVORED

I was teaching about primary health care in the community and had students in a number of agencies, such as Head Start, a women's shelter, and a homeless clinic. There was a lot of poverty and life-depressing situations in which people were living. But this is a funny story. I had a couple of students that were doing home visits with a Head Start teacher in a rather poor section of Cincinnati. Following their clinical hours in the morning, we would gather in the afternoon to discuss the events of the morning.

One student related that the home she visited was very roach infested. The mother was using the child's doll to hit the roaches as they ran around the table. Then the child would hold the doll for a bit, then the mom would take it and hit a few more roaches. Certainly this environment was very different from the lives our students were living.

That evening around the dinner table she shared her experience with her family. They wanted her to quit the nursing program and stated this was no place for a young lady to be! That was in the early 1990s.

She prevailed in her studies, as nursing is not just about dealing with the poor. It was a good learning experience for the students, as they learned that not everybody lives in nice little suburban homes.

Patricia A. Slater, Petersburg, March 6, 2013

TAKING STUDENTS TO SENIOR CENTERS

I also used to take students to senior centers to do feet. That is very important for people who are elderly and diabetic. I usually had anywhere from six to eight students, and we would be greeted when we came into these senior centers by maybe sixty or seventy people lined up in chairs ready to have their feet taken care of.

Needless to say, by the time we were done the students had to go to two different places, one the first day and the next two days later. Going in the second time was difficult, for after they had experienced it once they were not in a hurry to go back to the second place! But then they had the nerve to ask me if I would take on the third trip, and I said, "You people are out of your mind," not that they had to go twice! [Laughter.]

But that was quite a learning experience because you are confronted by people who could not care for themselves in certain aspects. As much as we don't like to do it, there are certain things that nurses don't want to do, things that nobody else would do.

Patricia A. Slater, Petersburg, March 6, 2013

ODD ASSIGNMENTS

I was hired at William Booth Memorial Hospital in Covington, Kentucky, soon after I received my BSN [bachelor of science in nursing] from Berea College. I always felt that I was an advocate for my patients. At one time that sort of seemed to get me in trouble. We were using a new kind of cancer treatment that required patients to stay in bed while a special pump infused their drugs intravenously.

I was the nurse in charge of my floor when I got a call from the admitting office that a woman was being admitted to bed one in a semiprivate room. When she arrived on my unit I sent someone to put her to bed. The patient requested to see me. This patient had been our patient previously for a series of cancer infusions. She knew that she would have to stay in bed the entire time. She asked me to get her transferred to bed two so that she would be able to look out the window.

Since her request seemed reasonable to me, I called the admitting office. I was told by the person in that office that they were too busy to be doing a transfer. When I explained that to the patient, she said, "Mrs. Smith, I can't be lying there by the door and seeing nothing for the next week or so. I have to be in bed two."

I called admitting again and the director said, "Well, if she doesn't like it, take her to see Colonel Skinner." So I put the patient in a wheelchair and took her to Colonel Skinner's office. He was the hospital administrator. I told the secretary that I needed to see the colonel. He came immediately out of his office and asked, "What is this all about?"

I told him our situation and he said, "Nurse, get back to your floor and I will call you." Soon I was called to come get my patient and admit her to bed two.

Not long after that I got a call from the director of nursing, saying, "Mrs. Smith, from now on do not take everything someone tells you so literally."

My patient got what she needed. I was glad that I advocated for her even if it caused a bit of trouble for me. On the plus side, Colonel Skinner remembered Nurse Smith as long as she was administrator of the hospital.

Clara Fay Smith, Erlanger, March 6, 2013

DECISION TO BECOME A NURSE

I chose to become a nurse for a number of reasons, and it was a last-minute decision, not something I had ever thought about. Education beyond high school was not something that was talked about in my family. Resources were scarce, although there was mention that if anyone would go to college it would be my brother, so that option was not an option. My only knowledge of nursing was that I had a cousin who was a nurse. As I was about to graduate I was confronted with what I was going to do.

A friend was going to go to St. Elizabeth School of Nursing. Knowing that I had to do something, I somehow decided to take the entrance test for nursing with my friend. In scoring very well, I guess I thought that was something I could do. In those days women were usually directed toward going to college to be teachers, or you went to some kind of secretarial school, or got married and had children.

For me, after talking with my cousin and learning that nursing school was not too expensive, after the first year I decided to enroll. After making the decision, I entered St. Elizabeth School of Nursing, located in Covington, in 1957 and graduated in 1960.

Patricia A. Slater, Petersburg, March 6, 2013

REQUIRED CLOTHING

I entered St. Joseph School of Nursing as a seventeen-year-old after graduating from a small high school. Within weeks we began to understand that the next few years would be a challenge. The school, being a Catholic institution, was at that time run predominantly by the nuns.

Stories abounded about the strictness of dress code. Shoes had to be polished and shoestrings had to be gleaming white. It seemed that every nun, from the director of the school to those in the hospital, [was] on the lookout for a scuffed shoe or a dirty shoestring.

There was even a rumor that a few years prior to my time students had to line up each morning before going to their units and be inspected, not only for clean shoes and shoestrings but clean caps and well-pressed uniforms. Since the hospital laundry did our uniforms, that was not too much of a problem

Patricia A. Slater, Petersburg, March 6, 2013

Nurse's First Patient

I remember my first patient. We had learned the procedure of giving a bed bath in the lab and had practiced and received a passing grade from our instructor. It was now time to go to a hospital and do a complete bath on a real person. Anxiously we walked over the bridge from the dorm to the hospital unit to which we were assigned. Our fears were mounting, wondering if we could really do this. We waited as she gave each one their assigned room number.

She came to me, gave me the room number, and informed me that it was a male patient who was sixteen and had a gunshot wound in the leg. I was mortified and wondered, how could this be? I didn't know how to converse with someone of the opposite sex that I didn't know, much less give him a bath. Thankfully, the unit had orderlies, so we were spared having to do the complete bath.

Being so challenged after passing the test, I knew I would succeed with all future patients.

Patricia A. Slater, Petersburg, March 6, 2013

The Way Things Were Back Then

Health care costs of today have escalated to cover the costs of modern technology, while at the same time direct patient care has been reduced, leaving much to be considered. The medical community blames it on the government. The government blames it on inappropriate care by the medical community. The patient lies confused someplace in between. Back then, the patient was at the forefront, and there is some nostalgia associated with that fact.

The first year we did douches, enemas, and TPR (temperature, pulse, and respiration) checks and patient ambulation. We learned to give medications, including intramuscular and subcutaneous injections, during the last part of the freshman year. We practiced on each other rather than an orange. We were told that you "couldn't get the real feel with an orange!" I am sure that was a true statement. The nursing instructor was brave enough to let me practice on her.

We had all the food we could eat in the hospital cafeteria. An experience that has remained funny to me throughout the years happened when our St. Joseph Hospital class was being oriented. The hospital dietitian came over to speak to us and welcome us to St. Joseph Hospital. He said, "We want you to feel at home. If there is any food that we can prepare for you, please let me know."

I quickly and eagerly raised my hand. He acknowledged me, so I told him that I would like cabbage pudding. He said that he didn't believe he had ever heard of that one. In retrospect, I can't recall the cabbage pudding (scalloped cabbage) ever being prepared for us at St. Joseph Hospital.

Evelyn Pearl Anderson, London; reprinted from Anderson,
Daylite's A-Comin' (Baltimore: Publish America, 2007), 47

INTERESTING BEGINNING YEAR

We did not have to go far [to our quarters], since the nurses' residence was alongside the hospital with a walkway in between. The nurses' residence was a different world for me, as some of the girls smoked, some used foul language, and some danced. These were all taboo for me in my growing-up years.

The rules at home were good and helped me be capable. However, I was ill-prepared for what was going on before my very eyes. The two girls next door and my roommate smoked, laughed, and talked most of the night. This definitely was not a lifestyle to which I was accustomed.

In November 1957 I became ill with the Asiatic flu. I was given the immunization, with a near-immediate response! I was quickly admitted as a hospital patient with this horrible flu, manifested by elevated temperatures to 103 degrees. I was hospitalized for nearly one week. Once I began feeling better, it was fun having visits from the mountain boys who were students at the University of Kentucky.

This hospitalization took a toll on my academic situation. At the end of the first semester I was on academic probation at the University of Kentucky. I am not sure that I understood exactly what that meant, because I was still eligible to go through the nursing capping ceremony. Capping was a very major event in the life of a young student nurse and represented her successful completion of the first semester of nurses' school and a large step towards the real thing. It was really a big deal to get to wear a white cap (no stripes the first year).

Through the years my mother kept my 1958 yearbook, *The Nightingale* from Good Samaritan Hospital School of Nursing. Within the pages are included wonderful pictures of my first-year class, where each student nurse was dressed in her uniform that had crisp white and blue sleeves, bodice, back, and sides. The sleeves had crisp white cuffs.

Evelyn Pearl Anderson, London; reprinted from Anderson,
Daylite's A-Comin' (Baltimore: Publish America, 2007), 18–19

Use of Last Names Only

It was around this time the national debate in nursing had begun, with discussions about nursing as a profession. The National League of Nursing sent representatives to St. Joseph's to evaluate the nursing programs. On one of those afternoons, Sister Jane Miriam stopped me in the front lobby and said, "Miss Carpenter, those NLN people aren't very happy with me for accepting the four of you. Miss Carpenter, you aren't going to let me down, are you?"

I said, "No, Sister, I will never let you down." And I didn't!

The use of our last name was the correct professional way to address a person. So it was "Miss Carpenter," "Miss Wells," "Miss Ritchey," and so on. We were not permitted to tell a patient our first name. My nametag read, "Miss P. Carpenter." The patients were always trying to guess what the "P" stood for. I don't recall anyone ever guessing "Pearl," but I do remember one person guessing "Penelope."

I found that to be amusing, but of course the real fear was that some patient from your hometown would call you by your first name. To prevent that, I would quietly caution the patient against using my given name. They found that very funny. It was strange that I was a nineteen- or twenty-year-old with sixty-plus-years-old [patients] calling me "Miss Carpenter."

Now I am a sixty-plus-year-old with nineteen- to twenty-year-olds calling me "Pearl." I suppose it is social change rather than a lack of respect.

Evelyn Pearl Anderson, London; reprinted from Anderson,
Daylite's A-Comin' *(Baltimore: Publish America, 2007), 43–44*

BECOMING A NURSE

When I was twenty-two years old I was still trying to get my act to-gether and decide what I was going to do with my life. I had taken a gap year and went to Belize with Raleigh International and lived in Cyprus the rest of the year. Then I had a very unsuccessful stab at the University of Durham and had dropped out during the first semester, as I could not imagine how studying the classics and English were going to help me get a practical job in the real world, unless I was going to consider being a teacher. Having a special-needs teacher as a mother, I had long ago been told the challenges of this profession, so that was clearly not the right avenue for me, so I started waitressing. I guess I hadn't really stopped since my first job wearing a dreadful straw hat and green pinstriped waistcoat, serving fish and chips and cups of tea on Scarborough's beachfront at age thirteen. It just became a full-time occupation. I scouted the paper on a regular basis looking for "the job." At that point I was very much against going back to the university. I thought, a person can get a job without a degree these days; thus that was the stubborn stance I took. My mother deserved an award for her patience putting up with me.

So I landed an interview and got a job as a nursing assistant on an orthopedic floor of a very posh private hospital—the Bournemouth Nuffield Hospital. I was very perturbed to have to wear an ugly brown dress and, having never worked in health care before, I had a very star-tling first day. I got teamed up with another nursing assistant and off we start[ed], gathering linen to change the patient's beds. I thought it was all going rather well when putting nice, clean sheets on the beds; then one of the nurses asked me to help one of the patients to the bathroom. So I helped the lady to the commode, handed her the call bell, and hurried away, slightly embarrassed. The embarrassment deepened when I then had to help the lady off the commode and actually wipe her bottom. I don't know what I expected, as it was obvious I had not thought the job through properly. That was terrible, since I had to wipe a complete stranger's bottom.

The girl I was teamed up with found this terribly amusing, and she also taught me to see the funny side when she said, "We see it all here—bottoms, willies, everything, and you haven't seen anything yet!" And so I continued working as a nursing assistant and began to realize that if I didn't pursue it further I would regret it. So I swallowed my pride and admitted to my mother that perhaps she was right after all, so I signed up at Bournemouth University for my BSN in nursing.

Being a student nurse could be a story all in itself. I remember numerous times that I passed out and humiliated myself with the sometimes shocking events that I witnessed, such as a limp, lifeless toddler in the emergency room getting her shinbone drilled for osseous emergency access. However, sometimes just the early morning start would be enough for me to just keel over and land on my face while the nurses were trying to give report. Everyone would tell you to take full advantage of being a student and "go see everything." So seeing your first knee operation, no one tells you how graphic it actually is until it is too late. The sight of someone's bone and the smell of cauterized skin is clearly too much for me. I learned I was not cut out for surgery after waking up on a trolley with an oxygen mask on, right next to the patient, also seeing the baby being born for the first time, or seeing a C-section, where the doctor just reaches into the woman's stomach and a pink, slimey mess of a beautiful baby suddenly appears.

Some coworkers would offer reassurance with words like, "Don't worry, love," and "It happens to the best of us." Others would be more critical by saying, "So you're going into nursing?"

Louise Webb, Bowling Green, June 10, 2013

NURSING SERVICES IN ENGLAND

During my last year of studies I happened to answer an e-mail regarding a foreign exchange opportunity for nursing students to go to America, with accommodations and food to be reimbursed, and the chance to see how nursing differed stateside [it] was the opportunity of a lifetime. Nursing is wonderful in that the same principles apply no matter what country you choose to work in; the goal is the same, to be there for the patient. However, there are many different cultures of nursing. For example, the English culture of nursing in the National Health Service has a certain dress code, which requires nurses to wear tunic tops with trousers or a dress to work. Also, a nursing watch pinned to your uniform is a requirement. There were no *Grey's Anatomy* scrubs, dangling earrings, or chewing gum offered.

In England patients usually expect to be roomed in a bay housing, at least six patients with nothing more separating the beds than a thin, ancient curtain that has been around since the 1930s. Only if you are contagious to other patients [are you] given the luxury of a private room, unless you can afford private health insurance. You live in fear of the ward sister or matron, or at least I remember being fearful of the "boss lady," as woe betide you if a doctor reports you for not following orders or a patient has a complaint.

I miss the tea breaks, since there was always a plentiful supply of tea to sustain you through a shift, but I have learned to love coffee stateside.

Louise Webb, Bowling Green, June 10, 2013

English Nurse's First Work in America

My first experience of nursing in America was simply fantastic. Six people all total were selected for the trip. The two destinations were North Carolina and Bowling Green, Kentucky. We all flipped a coin to decide where we would go. It was amazing, the twists and turns of fate in life, as that coin landed me in Kentucky, where I met my wonderful husband eight years ago. My mother jokingly warned me not to meet an American just before I headed for America.

Eight months after the exchange, Craig got his first passport and survived a flight to England to ask permission to marry me. He later told all the new people we met that I was his first mail-order bride! Anyhow, I spent twelve weeks rotating [through] different clinical sites in Kentucky and had a huge variety of experiences.

I got to work in the nursery, the ICU, and the med-surg floors. They even allowed me to ride in the medivac helicopter to see if I would like to be a flight nurse. Then they took us to the country and we got to see what home-health nursing was like in rural Kentucky and in an Amish community. Patients that spring to my mind at that time include an Amish man with a huge aneurysm. He had been diagnosed with a dissecting aortic aneurysm and was told that he needed immediate surgery or else he was risking death.

He had decided to come home and pray about it. He told us that happened while he was strapping a heavy plough onto one of his workhorses so that he could continue plowing his fields. He had the attitude of "what will be, will be." He did not have insurance, and he did not want his community to combine their funds to help him, as they usually do for health needs.

Louise Webb, Bowling Green, June 10, 2013

Coping with the Unexpected

The twelve weeks of my exchange event went by so fast. I returned to England to finish my degree. I then went through many hurdles and life curveballs and it felt like moving heaven and earth to transfer my nursing degree from England to America after I got married and moved to Bowling Green. A tortuous and stressful eighteen months total, and I think doctors from foreign countries must have some sort of speed-dial system and have a far easier time of it.

Being a new nurse in a new nursing culture where you could wear comfy scrubs was both exciting and completely terrifying at the same time. Fresh out of school is when you stop and realize that perhaps you are only just beginning to learn what nursing is really all about. It is beyond stressful, and you feel an overwhelming responsibility towards the patient. Especially when it is 3:00 a.m. and your patient is suddenly taking a turn for the worse and you have to get on the phone and wake the doctor up and get shouted at on the phone in some situations. Actually the problem could have waited, but you are so worried, being a new nurse. You need reassurance about any slight variation from the expected.

Louise Webb, Bowling Green, June 10, 2013

Nurse-Doctor Relationships

I still remember the feeling of terror in the pit of my stomach whenever I had to talk with one certain doctor. But now, with perspective, I can clearly see that most doctor-nurse relationships are well established and functional, yet at the same time I was not convinced that this certain doctor was [not] vindictive and enjoyed making me feel as stupid as he could.

I would bring to his attention that a patient's urine output was very low after surgery; then he would enjoy letting me know in front of everyone at the nurses' station that this was entirely my fault.

Another time, with a patient going downhill, I dared to call him on a Sunday afternoon and was puzzled that he was answering the phone with a whisper and would quickly give me an order and then hang up.

I found out on my third phone call that I was disturbing his deer hunting, and he then said, "Please stop calling me and start doing your job properly so that the patient will not be having this problem."

Louise Webb, Bowling Green, June 10, 2013

DAY SHIFTS VERSUS NIGHT SHIFTS

Nurses need a lot of support, both hands-on support from nursing assistants and emotional support from their peers. This is especially true for new nurses, and one confounding problem that I actually witnessed was nurses "eating their young," which is a term used for giving the new nurses a really hard time. Hopefully this is not commonplace, and from what I recollect it appears to take a good manager to become aware of the problem and stamp it out.

New nurses are usually given the night shift to work at first, until they become more seasoned and experienced to be able to cope with the busier day shift. So giving report to the day-shift nurse was the time most dreaded. It seems the decisions you made during the night were "stupid," and you were made to feel that you were ruining the day-shift nurse's day already because she was going to have to fix all the things you had left undone. In reality, nursing is a twenty-four-hour-a-day job, since it is a continuous cycle of care. You have to hand over tasks to the next shift, because if you stayed to do them you would never get to go home.

Louise Webb, Bowling Green, June 10, 2013

CHANGES ACROSS THE YEARS

Way back in the 1960s, when I became a registered nurse, things were a lot different. Intravenous fluids came in glass bottles with screw tops and patients' arms were taped to arm boards because the only available needles were metal and unbending. Respiratory therapists had not been invented. Physical therapists were in their baby stages. Dieticians were available a few days a week for consultation only for hospital menus.

Pharmacists were in their own pharmacies, making money, and usually visited the hospital weekly. In other words, the nursing staff members did everything, and quite well, I might add.

So here I enter this scene as a recent graduate from one of those new four-year nursing programs, as green as grass. Unlike the popular diploma schools of nursing, my education had been on theory and principles, with minimal clinical experiences, based on the premise that, given the knowledge, I could rapidly gain the skills with experience, and I did do just that!

Theresa Sue Milburn King, Danville, June 18, 2013

Saying Goodbye to the Patient

I was working at a clinic in Kentucky and there was this young male that complained of right-sided abdominal pain. At the time, the doctor I worked for had two of us working with triaging patients. The young man was guarding his abdomen because the pain was intense. The doctor went in to see him and ordered a complete blood count. We sent the patient to the lab on this Friday afternoon, and with this test it comes back within twenty minutes or so. The test came back showing this patient had infection in his body. He was hurting in his lower-right part where the appendix is located.

So the doctor calls the hospital to see if he could fast track the patient, because it was possible he had appendicitis. As the patient was leaving and holding his abdomen, the girl that was working with me says to the patient, "Have a good weekend."

That was just a habit we always say when the patient exits. It is something to the fact of having a good day. Well, she said, "Have a good weekend" when the patient was going to the hospital with possible appendicitis.

Dana Burnam, Bowling Green, July 29, 2013

Missouri Nursing Facility

I had the experience of being the first registered nurse consultant at a Missouri nursing home housed in what had once been the Polk County Poor Farm Home. This was a very new idea, for nursing homes to have a consultant, and a very new idea for me to even consider. I would go out to the home every week to talk with the nurse's aides about any and all aspects of patient care. I found that I became very excited about diagramming and explaining the functions of a Foley catheter or any other part of patient care issues.

I still remember the sparkle of excitement in the eyes of an older nurse's aide as she learned there really was a purpose in the Foley catheter, along with the anatomy involved with the insertion and subsequent care.

It was here that I learned to stand on my own two feet professionally. The owners of the nursing home, who were nonmedical and nonprofessional, had opened some rooms for about six mentally retarded patients from the Nevada, Missouri, hospital. The reason to accept these persons was to be part of a pilot program to see how the mentally retarded would function in a more homelike environment.

Another function of mine as a consultant was to assist in the preparation of nutritionally correct menus, and this I did. On Thursdays I would drive through a cornfield and pull up by the side of the house. While getting out of the car I would smell the most wonderful aromas coming from the kitchen. I felt so proud that I had had a part in the meal planning and had satisfaction in knowing that the patients were receiving nutritionally correct meals.

There was a large cornfield next to the lawn of the personal care home. During a fall afternoon one of the new residents left the building without anyone knowing that he did. I am not sure how long he had been missing before someone noticed he was gone. An immediate search was begun and some neighbors were called in to canvas the cornfield with tall corn standing in it. After an hour or so they found him in one of the rows of corn. Needless to say, after that a better watch for him was kept. I suspect the resident was relieved to get . . . out of the endless maze of tall corn.

Evelyn Pearl Anderson, London, July 18, 2012

8

Doctors and Nurse Interns

Very few accounts about doctors and nurses serving as interns were provided. Most of the following stories are informative, telling about such things as the importance of mothers, slow-learning medical and servant processes, the crucial role of horses for transportation purposes, and erroneously performing services on a dead body prior to the doctor's arrival to pronounce the person dead.

Mother's Importance

I was on the elevator with several medical students and asked one of them who was the most important person in their time as a medical student and who could make them or break them. One of the medical students took an interest in my question, and I quickly told him that a nurse should be the most important person.

He informed me that his mother was a nurse, at which point I informed him that I had no doubt he had been brought up right.

Jo Ann M. Wever, Springfield, March 14, 2012

Nurses Don't Wait on Doctors

In July new medical interns and residents start rotations at the medical center. I was talking to another nurse when a new intern came up to us and asked for several items. The other nurse and I looked him up and down, then she said to me, "He has no broken arms."

I said, "He has no broken legs," and then we told him where he could get the items he needed.

He turned red in the face and headed in the direction that we had told him to go. The lesson we hoped he learned was that we do not wait on doctors.

Jo Ann M. Wever, Springfield, March 14, 2012

FEARFUL SURGERY RESIDENT

Late one night a surgery resident who had come to see one of my patients asked me to walk him to the elevator. I told one of the other nurses that I would be back shortly. The elevator was near the waiting room, where many family members of patients slept.

The resident was small in height and slim. I never knew why he wanted me to walk him to the elevator. I am five feet and nine inches tall and have never been accused of being slim or small in stature. I could only guess that he wanted me to protect him from something or somebody.

Jo Ann M. Wever, Springfield, March 14, 2012

INITIAL SERVICE AS A COURIER

I was terribly shy when I first came here [Frontier Nursing Service area]. I listened more than I talked. But there was continuous talk about how you could cope with the problems of that center on the way home. Oh, yes! And Mrs. Breckinridge would tell you about these people. She would tell about their contribution to help build the center. She also talked about some of the problems. So you began to become closely aligned with them as you talked to them, and Mrs. Breckinridge very definitely did it.

That all happened during the first two weeks I was here. They had more nurses than couriers in those days, so she asked me if I would like to come to Wendover to work as a courier for a couple of weeks. Naturally, that was a very good way to break me in, and I hadn't ridden horses for a while. I rode them back in Texas, sitting in a western saddle. Well, I started getting used to riding them in the mountains, something I had never done before. . . .

I was at Wendover for three weeks doing courier work. It was very important to take good care of your horse, because that was your sole means of transportation.

Told by Gertrude Isaacs to Dale Deaton, November 15, 1978;
provided by the Louie B. Nunn Center for Oral History,
University of Kentucky Libraries, Lexington

After a Patient Dies

Something that was funny about my nursing school experience happened when we were seniors and were appointed to be in charge of a unit. Of course, the registered nurse in the area was always watching and helping us out. My teammate and I had a patient one night who died. We knew what to do when a patient died, such as what procedures were to be done to care [for] the body of the deceased.

We went in and straightened the bed out and straightened the patient out, turned his oxygen off, put his false teeth in, and got him prepared to be turned over to the mortuary. So when we went back out to the nurses' desk, a nurse's aide said, "Oh, you're not supposed to do all that; you are supposed to wait until the doctor comes and pronounces him dead."

So what did me and my friend do? We went back into the room, rolled him back up, turned the oxygen back on, took his teeth back out, so as to have him as he was when he died!!

That was sort of crazy for us to do, but we thought at the time that must be what we were supposed to do. Nothing was ever said about what we did, but to us, years later, it was rather funny.

Told by Martha Hill, Glendale, to Mark Brown, June 30, 2012;
provided by the Kentucky Historical Society, Frankfort

At Nursing School

I always felt like I was behind. I started out in a diploma program at St. Elizabeth School of Nursing in Covington, and by the time I finished they said, "Well, you ought to have a degree from a college." So a few years later I went and got a degree in psychology from the University of Cincinnati. Then they said, "Well, you need a degree in nursing." So I waited a few more years and then went and got a degree in nursing from Northern Kentucky University, and after I finished the baccalaureate they said, "Well, you really need a master's." So I went and got a master's degree, and when I finished with that I started teaching. They said, "Now, if you want to stay teaching, you've got to get a PhD." I started on the PhD, and then I said, "Now, wait a minute."

At that time I was going to be teaching only a few more years, and then I said, "You can send me on my way and I'll do something else, or you're going to put up with me without a PhD." I taught for a few more years, and I was ready for retirement.

Patricia A. Slater, Petersburg, March 6, 2013

On Call, 1960

During my second year, we worked medical, surgical, and orthopedics. During this time we administered medications, which we all looked forward to doing. The time came when I didn't really like to give medicines. We were taught to administer intravenous (IV) solutions, but we were never to administer blood or blood products. A medical doctor was the only medical team member permitted to administer blood. The IV solutions were in glass containers.

If seated in the nurses' station, charting, and a physician walked in, we student nurses and graduate registered nurses were to stand immediately and proceed to hand the physician his (rarely a female) patient's charts. Failure to stand would result in a reprimand. We would then accompany the physician to his patient's room and assist as needed.

There were stories of doctors being disrespectful to nurse/nursing students. Thankfully, I never had that problem.

Evelyn Pearl Anderson, London; reprinted from Anderson,
Daylite's A-Comin' *(Baltimore: Publish America, 2007), 50–51*

Training Nurse's Aides

Due to new regulations back in the 1980s, all nurse['s] aides had to be suddenly certified by passing a state-maintained instructional program, with no exceptions. As a Medicaid nurse['s] aide instructor, one of my first classes was at a local county hospital. This group included all presently employed nurse['s] aides. I totaled up their collective years of previous experience as an aide and stopped when I reached 150 years.

Most of them resented this instruction in their lives. Written tests were given periodically. Consequently, I finally figured out one could not read, probably undetected by her employer, so I had to administer all her tests verbally.

One of the many class topics was bathing of a patient. The written test covered such things as safety and privacy issues and correct order of the best bed bath. And then there was the question, "What is a partial bath?"

Needless to say that I, as the instructor, was in shock and awe when I read one student's response as "tits and pits." While not completely correct, I decided to give full credit due to the originality and honesty of the answer.

By the way, that group of women was one of the best classes assembled.

Theresa Sue Milburn King, Danville, June 18, 2013

9

Various Types of Stories

Stories in this chapter are different enough that they need to be kept separate from other categories in this book.

Included are stories about the lack of suitable houses, discomfort caused by heat or cold, children who suffered from worms or a lack of quality drinking water or adequate food, makers of moonshine whiskey, hitchhikers, the return of nurses as supportive spirits, and the list goes on.

Unaccustomed to Summer Heat

When I first got to Hyden I worked in the hospital for a few weeks at what I seem to remember as relief work. I think I worked in practically ever[y] center, and I stayed in Confluence with Cherry Evans for quite a while. During the summer we liked to get up early because it was so hot. We liked to do our work in the mornings.

Cherry also came from England, so it was really just like an English setup. We'd have breakfast, then saddle the horses, and off we'd go to do our rounds. I think we'd take our lunch with us in sandwich form and then come back before it got too hot in the afternoon. We worked in certain clinics, such as Hell for Certain and Confluence. Cherry also had one up in Grassy.

The homes were mostly clean and tidy; thus the ones that were pretty poor stood out like a sore thumb. There was one home in Hell for Certain that had no windows, only one door, and the family lived in this house without a toilet. I don't know how they lived. They were just like rabbits! I thought that was quite unusual.

Told by Lydia Thompson to Carol Crowe-Carraco, 1978;
provided by the Louie B. Nunn Center for Oral History,
University of Kentucky Libraries, Lexington

DAILY HOME SERVICES

When we made house calls we rode on a horse to give shots, inoculations and things. When we got there we were always asked in and we were always offered water to wash our hands with. We were treated with respect when we got there.

One of the most common ailments with children were worms. We tried to dose them regularly for worms, but the manifestations were really quite appalling. Kids would also have symptoms of pneumonia and appendicitis, and if it had gone too far we couldn't dose them until the condition had subsided. The routine practice was to dose them twice each year.

People there lived where there was water to drink, so I don't think they drank the river water [which could be a source of worms]. When they were looking for a place to build their home, they'd find water first and then build their home around it.

Told by Lydia Thompson to Carol Crowe-Carraco, 1978;
provided by the Louie B. Nunn Center for Oral History,
University of Kentucky Libraries, Lexington

MISS BRECKINRIDGE, NOT COUSIN MARY

I was a junior courier [in the FNS] during the summer [of] 1959, and it was mostly fun. We'd get up in the mornings and go to breakfast, then we would help with the horses. After that we would take a picnic lunch and go down to the river and paddle around in a boat. We would help put the horses out in the morning and we would help bring them in at night, including the mule.

We would go horseback riding in the evening after dinner, but one of the functions that we did was fix tea. We also helped Miss Breckinridge gather the eggs. Since Carlyle Carter called her Cousin Mary, Miss Breckinridge requested that I also call her Cousin Mary, but it was very difficult and it didn't last very long. I always kept saying "Miss Breckinridge" when I should have been saying "Cousin Mary." However, since she wasn't my cousin, I just couldn't get into it.

Told by Carrie M. Parker to Dale Deaton, September 29, 1979;
provided by the Louie B. Nunn Center for Oral History,
University of Kentucky Libraries, Lexington

Community Garbage

Stinnett was part of my district, and up past it was another hollow that had a [creek] branch that went up, but not very far. It was called Greasy, and it was really a beautiful place. There was a family on the mouth of that [creek] where I wouldn't treat their children because of worms until they built their toilet. That kind of thing was the only way we had so as to treat.

The other thing that we all did in those days was to squash garbage. We didn't always have very many canned foods. In those days it was really bottled foods, but we squashed the cans down flat and buried them in a big hole in the ground and then laid boards on top of the hole. We tried to teach this to people in the district, but they didn't catch on very well, and that's why we see so much garbage along here now.

It's really hard to know how much of an impression we made on them. It was Mrs. Breckinridge's idea that the local people should dig holes and then put garbage in the holes.

Told by Molly Lee to Eliza Culp, February 6, 1979;
provided by the Louie B. Nunn Center for Oral History,
University of Kentucky Libraries, Lexington

Food and Children

I don't think we ever did much in the food line. It's very hard to change a culture that has almost grown up with the bare necessities of life that [were] seldom available. The ones who did not work did not feed. They were the ones who were either lazy or too ill-nourished to work, perhaps in poor health. There were not very many persons that had tuberculosis at Beech Fork back then, but for some reason they couldn't dig a garden and put their backs into it. However, they always had pigs and chickens.

All of them had large families and worked very hard. Kids also worked in the fields. They didn't eat beef in here for years, so what they had to eat was pork and chicken.

Back then children were very useful in gardening and field work activities, and a great number of them helped with the hoeing. It depended entirely on how well organized the family was. The children were very much a workforce in all ways. The older girls would help with the housework, and back then, when there were large families, the older kids brought up the younger ones.

*Told by Molly Lee to Eliza Culp, February 6, 1979;
provided by the Louie B. Nunn Center for Oral History,
University of Kentucky Libraries, Lexington*

A NIP OF MOONSHINE WHISKEY

One of the things I learned as a young person is that there are three things I do not know about, and they are religion, politics, and alcohol. I'm a past master at not getting involved in those subjects. Speaking of alcohol, revenuers were gone by the time I got here, but there were still many people who made their own whiskey or who did bootlegging. One of the things that we were told was that you never know where a still is. But when I went on district work I decided right fast that the best way I could stay out of problems was to know where stills were and then to look the other way. We got questions from local people as to our feelings about alcohol. As a matter of fact, when I was at Red Bird one of the men put a still in, and to avoid going past his still when making a house call was a half hour or half mile wide. I would have to go around his still, then on up the hill. Since it was so far around, I went to see the man and said, "Look here. I want to go up that path that goes down by the creek at the foot of the hill."

He said, "Well, what day do you want to go on?"

I said, "Wednesday afternoons." Then he said, "All right, if you go up there and always look to the left as you're going up and look right when coming down you can go up on Wednesday afternoons."

So he had bouldered up the place across the path so you wouldn't get to it, and every Wednesday at noon it was down and I rode my horse. I looked this way going up and looked this way coming down. I always knew where the stills were. They used to make good liquor, but I don't think they do anymore. I always knew where the stills were, so this is a good place to mind your own business!

I had one family that used to put up three new barrels of whiskey every fall, and every fall they took off three barrels of whiskey and gave away one of them. The other two barrels were for their medical purposes, and one year I was going to go up to see my family and my brother, who had never tasted moonshine whiskey. So they gave me a half gallon to take up to my brother.

At that time, on rare occasions when I went to Wendover and had sherry, that was about as much as I ever drank. And one time up at Beech Fork I had been out most of the night and had also worked hard all day. So at 10:00 p.m. I got called for midwifery, and it was about five o'clock in the morning when I was ready to go home, but they had fixed some breakfast for me. Of course, you know that I was really out on my feet. Well, this man fixed coffee for me, and he laced it well! I do know I went to sleep on my horse going home, but as far as I know that's the only time I ever tasted liquor in the district.

He didn't even ask if I wanted it, he just knew I needed it.

When I went back to see this woman the next day she told me what her husband had done. I said, "No wonder I went to sleep on my horse."

She then said, "Well, he followed you down to see that you got home all right."

Told by Grace Reeder to Carol Crowe-Carraco, January 25, 1979;
provided by the Louie B. Nunn Center for Oral History,
University of Kentucky Libraries, Lexington

Serving Students

Back when I was out on service in [the Red Bird area] there were a lot of one-room schoolhouses, and I would go around and give the immunizations and go around and see the children in the schools. In doing that I would bring them a Bible lesson as well as give them their shots, and we'd just have a good time and also have lunch together. It was really a home-type atmosphere, but they'd have as many as eight grades of students in one schoolroom. They had no books, or at least very few. Most of the books were old and worn out and not up-to-date at all. The teacher usually had maybe one or two years of college at most. They loved the kids but were more of a babysitter than a teacher.

When consolidation came along it was extremely difficult for people to get used to, because when you think about a little six-year-old having to walk out to the main road way before light comes in the morning. They might not get home until four or five o'clock in the afternoon, because if they were the first ones picked up they would be the last ones dropped off. That was a long day for those little children, so it really was hard. But they got used to it, and a lot of families moved closer to the main road.

There were a lot of school days missed back in those old days. The education process wasn't very good because they didn't have any supplies or preparation for it. However, a few children from the Red Bird area went to high school, but high school was mainly for the city kids.

Told by Elsie Maier to Dale Deaton, December 5, 1978;
provided by the Louie B. Nunn Center for Oral History,
University of Kentucky Libraries, Lexington

A MIDWIFE IN KENTUCKY

While [I was] serving as a midwife in England, Miss Cashmore called me and said they needed a midwife in Kentucky. I can remember saying, "Kentucky? What's that?" I didn't really know much about American geography. Anyway, she said that she would like, if possible, for me to come and talk to her about this as soon as I had finished with the case I was working. I went to talk with her before I went home and told her I had three cases booked ahead, then I said, "Well, they wanted somebody right away. I can't possibly go before June or July because I have commitments."

When she told me it was horseback riding in a rural area it sounded very exciting to me, so I said, "I'll think about it."

She said, "Well, I'll get application forms and one permission form and have them sent to your home." She did, so I applied for the [midwife] job and arrived here [in Kentucky] about six weeks later, in July 1938. . . .

I had been here for a year but I hadn't been out. After I had gotten here in July, Britain went to war in early September. And this is when the British nurses that were here suggested they had to go home. They had to go home, so they sent for me, because I was working at Hyden on the Bull Creek District, I guess. And I said I really would like a vacation, and then I was feeling a little bit hemmed in by the hills, so they said, "All right, but where are you going?"

I said, "Well, as far away as I can go. I'll go to Vancouver Island, where my mother has some cousins."

You paid anything in those days, but you didn't have anything to spend your money on. I can still remember to this day that the round-trip ticket from Lexington to Vancouver was $200, and it was tourist season. On the way out of here I was assigned a seat all to myself on the train. I couldn't believe it. You know, today you couldn't believe it. Anyway, there were two Scotswomen on the train who were just coming and saying, "We just want to hear you talk." I think they were homesick for Scotland.

Told by Helen E. Browne to Carol Crowe-Carraco, March 26, 1979;
provided by the Louie B. Nunn Center for Oral History,
University of Kentucky Libraries, Lexington

HUNGRY TIMES

I graduated from Cincinnati General Hospital, which meant that we had most of the poverty-stricken people that came in for service. And back then no one had any money, including the nurses. People are people wherever you find them. I did some private duty on what we called "Gold Coast." There were many things that you found that you had not seen before. People still got commodities. And in order to get flour, cornmeal, bacon, and lard, they had to also take grapefruit, and they got a whole sack of grapefruit but they didn't know how to use it. This one woman said, "We boiled 'em, we fried 'em. We tried everything, and we threw 'em over the hill and even the hogses [hogs] won't eat 'em." But then they were taught how to eat grapefruit and became accustomed to its tart taste and they loved it!

In a later period in my life, during World War II, we sent to Germany some cornmeal for the Germans to eat, but we didn't send cornbread recipes. And we sent them spoiled wheat to feed to their animals. Germans knew wheat but were not familiar with corn, so they used the spoiled wheat and boiled it even though it was mildewed and rusted and rotten sometimes, and they fed the corn to their cows and hogs.

A German exchange student spent some time with me when I was in upstate New York and we had cornbread. She said, "If somebody had only told us how to eat this, it's good, but we didn't know how to use it, so it was terrible. So we fed the good cornmeal, mixed it up with water and made slop out of it and fed it to our hogs. The cows liked it too!"

Told by Grace Reeder to Carol Crowe-Carraco, January 25, 1979;
provided by the Louie B. Nunn Center for Oral History,
University of Kentucky Libraries, Lexington

HITCHHIKERS

I remember one old gentleman who lived three or four miles up the creek above where we lived. He kept a granddaughter all the time, or she kept him. I'm not sure which, but this is a child, anyway, and she was sick one day. The grandfather decided to come to the clinic, but he had to walk most of the way until somebody stopped and gave him a ride.

He ended up being one of my in-laws and was quite an interesting old gentleman. He'd catch rides, which was another thing we did. We'd quite often give people rides. We'd be headed somewhere when somebody would stick their head in the side of the jeep and say or ask something, then ask, "Can I ride?"

We'd say, "Yeah, sure, jump in." There was never any thought of anyone harming one of the nurses.

Actually, we did have someone break in on us once, and I don't know for what reason they broke in other than he was drunk. It wasn't to steal, because my wallet was lying there and he didn't take anything.

Told by Jean Fee to Rebecca Adkins Fletcher, June 15, 2002;
provided by the Louie B. Nunn Center for Oral History,
University of Kentucky Libraries, Lexington

GETTING ADJUSTED TO THE COMMUNITY

There were a lot of problems in those days in keeping the road up, access road to the center, and maintaining a road so people could come in and go out. There were also problems like water supply, getting hay for your horses, and keeping enough nurses there to do the jobs that needed to be done. In those days [in the 1940s–1950s] the people were dealing with real concrete problems, like no telephones, didn't have a car or jeep, but you did have a horse. You were very dependent on the people around you, and I think they were very conscious of helping you. Whenever you came to the center back then and needed help you went to the local people for help. There was a very good community relationship you experienced back then when you came in as a new person. I think they were very favorable when accepting you as a new person, although one person always said, "Well, there are some good people and some not so good." I think they were cognizant of the difference between nurses. On the other hand, if they didn't like you very much they'd just tolerate you, sort of.

The committee meeting was a very important day for the community as well as for the nurses, because you did get to know the people better. As I say, "Bright eyed and bushy tailed." Of course, I was so brand new I was to the community just [a simple lady.]

I still remember those days very vividly.

Told by Gertrude Isaacs to Dale Deaton, November 15, 1978;
provided by the Louie B. Nunn Center for Oral History,
University of Kentucky Libraries, Lexington

Not Revenue Officers

Nurses rode horses around the mountains, but I never did it alone. I always went out with one of the nurses, and during our trip we were always told to sing at night so that revenue officers wouldn't think we were moonshiners and shoot us.

People made a lot of moonshine whiskey in the area, and people who were roaming around at night could be easily mistaken for revenue officers. So you sang endlessly at night.

Told by Anne Winslow to Anne Campbell Ritchie, September 25, 1979;
provided by the Louie B. Nunn Center for Oral History,
University of Kentucky Libraries, Lexington

Mary Breckinridge's Good Labors

The Frontier Nursing Services committees had trouble back then when trying to recruit younger people into the nursing service, and the committees also had to keep their fund-raisers going. Of course, the need for financial support is a little bit less since they've got more government financing now.

Mary Breckinridge certainly set [up] an amazing, extraordinary network of the committees and people. She had a lot of contacts with people she knew, or she knew other people who [helped set up] quite a network. And her family was very prominent, both politically and socially. Of course, she had contacts outside of Kentucky, so she knew how to make good use of those contacts.

Everybody talked about the time when she came up with a rubber ring after she had broken her back sometime between 1930 and 1933. After she came up we would go down to Wall Street in the subway, and she had on this huge rubber ring to sit on. She would say, "I'm Mrs. Breckinridge and I've got a broken back, so give me a seat, please."

Told by Anne Winslow to Anne Campbell Ritchie, September 25, 1979;
provided by the Louie B. Nunn Center for Oral History,
University of Kentucky Libraries, Lexington

HORSE OR JEEP

When I first went to eastern Kentucky I dare say there were horses at all the [FNS] centers, but even before I left there several years later most of the centers were getting along without horses because once people knew you had the jeeps you could go two or three different creeks each day as opposed to one creek a day. But I missed the joy of going out on horseback because you could see everything everywhere. You were out in the sun and it was beautiful, but you couldn't do anything like the load of work that you could now do by riding in the jeep.

Told by Mary Penton to Dale Deaton, June 15, 1979;
provided by the Louie B. Nunn Center for Oral History,
University of Kentucky Libraries, Lexington

FIRST IMPRESSION OF LOCAL FRONTIER NURSING

My first impression of [eastern Kentucky] was the dog that welcomed me most and took me up in the woods. There were not many people around, as it was dead between Christmas, which was over, and New Year's. It's hard to say what my first impressions were.

I very soon went to Wendover, and of course I was very excited about Wendover. There was a lady doctor here from the mission field and she did a [C-]section under local anesthetic. Also here was a nurse with whom I afterwards lived in Confluence. She was in the school as a student and she was very interested because I said, "Let's get the stretcher and go to the theater and pick up the patient there." It had been so long that I hardly knew if "stretcher" was the right word. What it did was getting the patient from the OR.

So I was able to watch the section under local anesthetic, which they were all done for years here. And then I helped clean a great big old-fashioned Isolette that we had. It was almost like a bathtub made of metal.

Well, that was one of the eye-openers in this small hospital in those days. They made do with very little. It was obsolete in most hospitals and would have been at this hospital but it kept babies warm and that was the thing it was supposed to do.

Told by Molly Lee to Carol Crowe-Carraco, February 6, 1979;
provided by the Louie B. Nunn Center for Oral History,
University of Kentucky Libraries, Lexington

BONZO THE PET PIG

Old Red L. Morgan lived up on Camp Creek out on the edge of the Frontier Nursing Service district. He was a bit odd. Anyway, one of the nurses had adopted an abandoned piglet. The sow had had a litter and she'd come along soon after, and this little piglet was abandoned on the hillside and the nurse decided to take it along for a pet. She named him Bonzo and taught him parlor tricks. She fixed him some dog food in a bucket and let him come in and stretch out in front of her fireplace in the cabin like a dog.

Of course, he grew up and got very mad if he didn't get his meals on time. He wanted dog food or human food, not pig food. He grew real tall and got to be rambunctious. I had to call the night watchman one night to get him [out from] in front of the cabin door because I'd gone to see Bucket, who was the assistant director, about some business. He came in and wanted to lie down in front of her fire, and Bucket knew I wouldn't want him to come in, so she didn't let him in. He got very mad, but then I said to Bucket, "Just call the garden house and tell them to ask the night watchman to come over and get the piglet away. I'm not going to leave this door as long as he's out there." Well, she did, and that was a great joke that went all over the service.

Soon after that, on a rainy day, Red L. came to the post office and he had with him $1.86 in his pocket, and as he went down to the turn in the road through Pig Alley he slipped and fell. Oh, Bonzo was running out there, and he came up and knocked Red L. down.

Likely claiming it was not Bonzo, Mrs. Breckinridge said that Red just tried to untie his shoestring but fell down.

Told by Agnes Lewis, Maryville, TN, to Dale Deaton, January 5, 1979;
provided by the Louie B. Nunn Center for Oral History,
University of Kentucky Libraries, Lexington

DOGS AT WENDOVER

I think we're all aware of the fact that dogs [breeds featured] by the American Kennel Club, first one dog and then another, become favorites of the American people. But when I first went down there [Wendover] they had these two beautiful large golden dogs, which I immediately recognized as something special. They looked just like big farm dogs to me, but I was informed they were golden retrievers from England and that this was a rare breed in the United States but that it was becoming popular in England. One of them belonged to Jean Hollins, who was a senior courier, and the other belonged to Miss [Dorothy?] Buck, one of the English nurses, a senior nurse. She had been a district nurse but was presently serving in administrative work.

The two dogs were Lizzie and Penny. Lizzie belonged to Jean Hollins and Penny belonged to Miss Buck, who was known as Bucket. They were magnificent dogs, as they were extremely friendly with everybody. I guess they were the spirit of Wendover at that time. They always flopped on the floor in front of the fire during teatime in the afternoon and nuzzled everybody. We didn't worry about washing our hands before we handed the cookies to ourselves or gave cookies to the dogs.

I think there have always been dogs at the Wendover tea event, and it kind of reminded me of the old English paintings in which you would always see the family gathered around the big fireplace, and there was always some kind of a dog in those pictures. Dogs were very much a part of Wendover firesides.

Told by Carolyn Booth Gregory, Evanston, IL, to Linda Green,
March 31, 1979; provided by the Louie B. Nunn Center for
Oral History, University of Kentucky Libraries, Lexington

STUDENT'S INCORRECT SPELLINGS

The nursing instructors always checked the content and student's spelling before letting them chart on the medical record. One day a freshman student wrote that she had left her patient in a semi-fowler's position. The position has the head raised about forty-five degrees and the legs barely raised behind the knees. When she got ready to chart, instead of putting that she had left her patient in a semi-fowler's position, she had spelled "semi-flour's" position.

I said, "I don't think that's what you want, you need to go back and correct that wording."

So she came back, and she had put it in a "semi-flower" position. She had to change it again and finally got it right.

It took her two or three times to get it spelled right, but at least it went on the records the right way.

Told by Martha Hill, Glendale, to Mark Brown, June 30, 2012;
provided by the Kentucky Historical Society, Lexington

The Roster Patient

A roster patient is one who does not have a physician, and usually the only rosters were in OB [obstetrics]. They had not sought a physician and maybe could not afford a physician to do their prenatal care. Usually when the physician did the prenatal care they would deliver the baby.

When these roster patients would come in and didn't have a doctor, they were assigned a doctor. Sort of like if you went to the emergency room, you would see a doctor who was working that night in the emergency room. The roster was actually a physician roster, more or less. They were assigned to certain patients during certain periods of time. When the rosters came in, the nurse would call that physician next on the on-call or roster list to come in to deliver the baby.

Told by Martha Hill, Glendale, to Mark Brown, June 30, 2012;
provided by the Kentucky Historical Society, Frankfort

Male Nursing Student's Failures

I guess the most stressful things that happen is when a student would do something unacceptable and was not going to pass the course. We teachers would probably be as concerned about it as the student was. That type [of] thing would be the most stressful event at the time, when the student would fail.

It was stressful to me wondering what kind of advice I could give that student in helping to pursue a nursing career. I remember one male student coming to school after getting out of the army, and he just didn't do well. He failed one course and so he was out for a semester or so, but he then reapplied and maybe passed that course but then failed the next course.

Finally I talked to him and said, "I'm not sure nursing is the career you should pursue." And it was stressful trying to guide him in another direction without him thinking we were just trying to get rid of him, because that wasn't the idea. He wasn't ever going to be successful in nursing, so he needed to think about something else.

I think he finally went into education and did fine.

That was the kind of stress I guess we had at times.

Told by Martha Hill, Glendale, to Mark Brown, June 30, 2012;
provided by the Kentucky Historical Society, Frankfort

FLY TUBES

This is a story about when I was working 11:00 p.m. to 7:00 a.m. shifts at the University of Kentucky Emergency Room, and since it was summer we had major fly problems. I had identified and reported the problem verbally, with no results. So one night I had to replace a suture tray that was being used to sew up a wound a patient had on his arm. Yes, a fly had landed on it. I decided that I had to do something to get the administrator's attention as to how serious [it was;] that flies anywhere in the hospital was not okay! I gathered up several handfuls of large test tubes and had a handful of incident reports and told the staff to kill any and all flies in the patient rooms and put them in the tubes and then have the doctor of that patient sign the incident report.

Of course, they all wanted to know what I was going to do, and [I] just said I would decide later; thus they got busy filling up test tubes. I regret that I didn't count the filled tubes and reports, although each fly got a report. At the end of the shift I collected the tubes and reports and had to put the tubes in a good-sized bag, and as I gathered our dead prey I decided what I would do.

I took the fly tubes and the reports to the acting administrator on our shift and explained our case to him and told him to put the flies in the tubes and the report[s] in piles on the head administrator's office desk. The acting administrator shook his head and said he would do it.

I was wakened up late afternoon when my supervisor called to tell me that for some reason there were workers all over the emergency room, and [they] were [working] on another set of doors. There were some electric things going up, so I said, "Great," and went back to sleep, since the problem was solved.

Jeri R. White, Lexington, July 1, 2012

CHILDREN'S SICKNESSES

I recall the child that had Rocky Mountain spotted fever. That was when I learned the sound of a central nervous system cry piercing down the hallways. It was a sound that I recognized again about five years later when cried out by my own youngest baby, enabling me to quickly respond.

Evelyn Pearl Anderson, London, July 18, 2012

COLD WINTER, 1961

The winter of 1961 arrived, and it was brutal. I lived in the nurses' residence, about one block from the hospital on the same street. It was high on a hill overlooking the Ohio River as it flowed from above Huntington, West Virginia, curving towards Cincinnati and beyond. Below and between was the city of Maysville, Kentucky. It seemed the winter's wind caught the cold moisture of the river's waters and blew its dampness furiously up onto the hospital hill.

I was very thankful for my cape that I had received from my parents during Christmas 1960, as it seemed to help me as I trudged on the one long, frigid walk to work.

Evelyn Pearl Anderson, London, July 18, 2012

A KILLING EVENT

There was a tragedy that happened while I was in Jackson, Kentucky. Miss Zilpha Roberts and other teachers had to go with their school trustees to meetings. This meeting was being held in Hazard, so Miss Roberts and the trustees went to Hazard to attend the teachers' meeting. Miss Roberts did not know there was a horrible feeling between two men in the community. One of the men said to the other man, "If you ever come up our creek and I meet you, I'll kill you."

The intended killing took place, and Miss Roberts was the only other person to see it when it happened. The man was not instantly killed, so he made them carry him across the field to his home. Well, then I took care of him. The feeling was strong that the man that lived across the creek from where Miss Roberts was teaching told her later that he feared for her life, thus sat on his porch with a gun across his lap, saying, "If the trees ever moved, I was going to shoot in the trees."

He was so afraid that the man would have somebody to kill her, so there would be no witnesses.

Well, that killing became known county-wide.

Told by Jean Tolk, Barbourville, to Dale Deaton, November 1, 1978;
provided by the Louie B. Nunn Center for Oral History,
University of Kentucky Libraries, Lexington

DEATH OF NURSE'S MOTHER

This is a personal story I am going to share with you. Twelve years ago I lost my mother of unknown causes. I had left my abusive husband and was at the police station filing an EPO [emergency protection order] due to the fact he had choked me the night before. My mother had taken ill and had been trying to call me to come home. She was watching my child, who was three years old at the time.

I got home and found her very ill, so we called the ambulance to come and take her to the hospital. I ran next door to get my sister to go to the hospital with my mom and dad. Needless to say, when I went to work the next day they called me in my office. I was the infection control nurse at the hospital. They said, "You need to come and talk to your mother because she is demanding to go home." I went to talk to her, and she was adamant about going home and sleeping in her own bed that night. The doctor let her go home because she told him that either he had to discharge her or she was going to walk out of here.

I went to stay with them that night with my four children because of the danger I was in with my husband. I helped her to the bathroom, and she laid her head on the wall and told me she was dying. Being her daughter and not thinking as a nurse, I told her it was the morphine they gave her and that it always made you act a little strange. At two o'clock that morning I could hear my dad calling for me in a panic, and when I got to their bedroom she was gone.

I started CPR until I collapsed. We never knew what happened to her, but for years to come I blamed myself for being a nurse and not being able to save my own mother. The words of my panicky father's voice rang in my head for years, until one day I finally understood that nurses are human and we can't save everyone.

Teresa Fryman Bell, Edmonson County, October 29, 2012

Smoking in a Wheelchair

A patient that had a stroke was sitting in a wheelchair at the nurses' station and was smoking a cigarette, which was allowed back then. He was also unable to speak very well as a result of the stroke. While he was smoking I looked over at him, and he was trying to get up and was making verbal sounds.

I told him he couldn't get up because he might fall and hurt himself. Suddenly I realized he had dropped the cigarette in his wheelchair and was trying to get up so as to not burn himself.

Jenny Burton, Bowling Green, May 8, 2013

Covered with Crabs

A young man was injured in a motorcycle accident, with multiple injuries. As a result of some of these injuries he was in traction. While I was making rounds one night he said to me, "I found a bug on me."

I picked it up and put in on a cloth and took it to the nurses' station in order to ask my fellow coworkers what they thought. We put it on a test tube and took it to the lab. While observing it under a microscope and watching the claws move, we decided it was a crab.

It turned out he was covered, so we moved his roommate out and then treated the young man by removing all the crabs from him.

Jenny Burton, Bowling Green, May 8, 2013

Potential Nurse Problems

When you first begin serving as a nurse, what do you do when you walk into an exam room and a patient is passed out, drunk, face down on the exam table, with their bottom hanging out of their jeans? What do you say when the patient tells you they accidentally walked into a broom and it lodged in their rectum? What do you do when a man is convinced he has a parasite roaming around his body and then starts shaking his head violently because he just felt it move around his brain?

A lot of situations I deal with by using my catchphrase[, which] includes, "Well, I'm just going to do a bit of research," or "I'll be right back in a minute," followed by a quick exit from the room and speed-dialing the attending doctor or asking my fellow NPs up the hallway.

So, for anyone reading this and possibly considering a career in nursing, I hope my commentary will inspire you to go for it, or at least have some compassion and respect for the very hardworking nurses that you may encounter in your life.

Louise Webb, Bowling Green, June 10, 2013

THE STORY OF MISS CHASE

Chase is the ghost that haunts the halls of Ephraim McDowell. She was supposedly a real person who worked as a nurse in the older portion of the hospital in the 1940s. She is said to continue watching over patients and roaming the hospital halls.

In an official McDowell [statement] written during the 1940s the hospital's one elevator at the time had a manual control, a far cry from the electronically powered systems in use today. Atop the old-fashioned elevator was an iron door that closed from the top down, thus keeping elevator patrons safely inside.

One day Nurse Chase, whose first name is unknown, entered the elevator but the iron door failed to come down and the elevator failed to move. Alarmed at this, Nurse Chase stuck her head out through the entrance to see what was going wrong. Without any warning, the iron door slammed down on Nurse Chase, instantly delivering a mortal wound. However, death apparently didn't prevent Nurse Chase from adhering to her nursing duties. For years she appeared to continue to aid hospital patients, with her spirit staying within the confines of the older section of the hospital.

Hospital employees working at McDowell in 1954 claimed to have experienced the ghost firsthand. One evening she was seen rocking a chair back and forth with no one else around it. One nurse said, "It did not bother me, because I knew Miss Chase was there. We always depended on her to help us. It was not uncommon for a nurse call bell to ring, and we would find a patient who had taken a turn for the worse. She was still watching over her patients."

A young girl who started working at the hospital in 1949 also experienced Nurse Chase. She said nurse call bells in patient wards would ring and the button for that room would light up, but there would be no one in the rooms when nurses went to check.

A former McDowell employee claimed to have worked with Nurse Chase both before and after the nurse's death. According to the hospital's history, this nurse was having trouble remaining awake at 4:00 a.m. during a night shift. She reportedly fell asleep in a chair but awoke when she felt a tap on her shoulder. No one was around her to do the tapping. She jumped up and checked on one of her patients in the pediatric ward and discovered the patient to be running a high fever.

Throughout the years Miss Chase's presence was often reported. Several nurses said they have felt the "swishing" of her starched uniform rushing by them in the hospital hallways. At one point a patient claimed to see Nurse Chase standing behind an actual nurse. On other occasions Miss Chase's white shoes were seen under privacy curtains.

In more recent times Miss Chase's appearances have tapered off. The old wing of the hospital is now used as office space, and Nurse Chase's presence seemed reluctant to move on to the newer portions of the hospital. One area she frequently haunted was the sixth-floor labor and delivery area where I worked night shift for almost fifteen years. I have felt and seen evidence of Miss Chase on numerous occasions, and while I did not feel fear at my experiences, it was a little eerie to be in the presence of something otherworldly.

The labor and delivery unit at Ephraim McDowell had an elevator that opened directly into the ward and required a key in order to operate. This elevator was mainly used by physicians and a handful of nurses who worked in the area. I lost count of the number of times I would hear the elevator "ding" and when the door opened up there would be no one there. Who operated the key to get the door open? We always blamed it on Miss Chase.

Near the elevator was a surgical sink, the type that must be opened by pressing your knee into a front level. At least once a month, sometimes more, this sink would turn itself on with no sign of anyone nearby. I would always have to walk down the hall in order to turn the sink off.

Because the labor and delivery unit had its own operating room for cesarean sections and tubal ligations, night shift was a time for us to restore the room with all the sterile equipment needed to get through the next twenty-four to forty-eight hours of work. The sterile supply room was downstairs on the second floor, and it was unusually quiet down there, with no one else around. I had a small wire cart I called my shopping buggy, and I would take it downstairs in order to be able to carry all the items back upstairs. Using my key, I would use the elevator, and it would open up into the sterile supply room.

One night after I had filled my buggy to capacity I was ready to head back upstairs. Pulling the buggy behind me, I was almost to the elevator when the buggy stopped moving. Thinking it had something stuck in the wheel, I tried pushing the buggy backwards, but it would not budge. It was like someone was holding on to the cart to keep me from moving it into the elevator. Spooked, I keyed the elevator and fled the second floor, leaving my buggy behind.

When I went back to the second floor I took someone with me and, you guessed it, the buggy rolled smoothly across the floor, making me look like a fool. However, I never went down to the sterile supply room by myself from that time until I finally left the hospital. I still believe Miss Chase was keeping me from moving that cart, but I do not know what the reason was.

The retired labor and delivery supervisor who had thirty-five years' experience said while she never experienced Nurse Chase personally during her personal tenure in the hospital, she's heard more than a few tales, all of which were about good things. My best friend and a retired nurse from Ephraim McDowell was a labor and delivery nurse who had experiences with Miss Chase. My friend said, "I lost the number of times a call bell would go off and there would be no one in the room, or the elevator would open up and there would be no one there. I definitely believe in Miss Chase, although I don't think she was out to hurt anyone. I think she was continuing to watch over her patients."

What I like to believe is that Miss Chase is watching over the patients at the hospital. I know people don't believe in these types of occurrences, but there were too many of them at Ephraim McDowell Regional Medical Center to be just a coincidence.

Bobbi Dawn Rightmyer, Harrodsburg, April 12, 2012

GHOST JOINED HORSE RIDERS

I loved to hear Betty Lester tell about some of the experiences she had as a district nurse. For instance, she can tell about various supernatural experiences that she had. One legend that she told us was about an area up the Thousandstick[s] Mountain located above the old hospital. She was coming through there one night and her horse stopped and refused to go any farther and then turned and bolted in the other direction.

She said that somebody told her long afterwards that no nurse was ever supposed to go through that section at night, because a local legend told by mountain people claims that somebody had been killed there and that if you came through there on your horse at night the ghost would jump up on your horse behind you and ride with you. No members of the Frontier Nursing Service believed that, but you just didn't flaunt the legends of the mountain people.

Well, Betty had not been told about this legend, and when she came through there and got to this section, her horse just bolted, because he didn't want to be ridden by a ghost! . . . It is said that back during [the early midwifery era] the nurses would never go anyplace alone after dark.

Told by Dorothy Caldwell, Burlington, to Marion Barrett,
January 18, 1979; provided by the Louie B. Nunn Center
for Oral History, University of Kentucky Libraries, Lexington

GEORGE'S GHOST

I was working second shift at a hospital and had for a long time. One particular night my nurse['s] aides, Maggie and Maudre, were putting their patients to bed and I was busy at the nurses' station, finishing up my nightly work. Out of the blue we heard a blood-[curdling] scream; . . . the girls were trying to put [a patient] back to bed, when they just dropped her quickly back into the chair and then came running out of the room and asked me if I was okay. I told them it wasn't me that screamed, that it was a patient in room 404-A. She was sitting straight up in bed when we went in to check on her. Then she asked us, "Did you see that man all dressed in white? He just climbed under my bed." We all were scared to death, so we searched the rooms and under all the beds.

Come to find out, when our patients saw George they soon died. The lady I had gone to check on died two days later.

See, George was a ghost that came with a patient to the hospital, and he would even whistle when we would go into her room. When she died, George stayed there with us, and we could hear him opening and closing drawers and closets, and we got so used to him we always welcomed him.

Teresa Fryman Bell, Edmonson County, October 29, 2012

HOSPITAL GHOST

In the hospital in which I worked we have a ghost that showed up from time to time and whose name was Irene. She did different things, like turn the call light on in an empty room, turn down the bed, turn lights on in an empty room, and made rockers rock, among different stunts. We had a photographer to take some photographs for an upcoming event, and in the photos from the nursery there was a mist seen in the corner, but only in these rooms.

There are several stories as to who she was and why she visited our hospital, but no one knows for sure. One story is that she lived on the property where the hospital was built and maybe died during childbirth, and that's why she liked to visit the nursery. Since the OB unit was closed, no one has heard from her since that happened, at least nothing about which I know.

Jenny Burton, Bowling Green, May 8, 2013

Hospital Workers and Patients

In this paper I have chosen to explore an aspect of what is found while working at a hospital during the so-called graveyard shift. This shift consists of the hours between eleven at night and seven in the morning. Working at night is very different from working during the day, especially when most of the people we are working around while they are asleep. I think this atmosphere is conducive to people's interactions, because they tend to be informal. Employees are relatively free to speak to one another, but there seems to be a degree of isolation involved in working at night, and the element of stress is forever present in a hospital and may make the employees need a form of release. This release may be in the form of storytelling, prank-playing, or just getting together to let off steam.

I chose this topic because I worked in the hospital for seven months as a nurse's aide and was quite familiar with the setting. Several of my friends still work there, and I didn't feel as if I would have any trouble gathering any information I might need. Most of my data was gathered through participant observation—things I remembered hearing or doing during the time I was employed at the hospital. I was able to obtain information from all over the hospital while I worked as a "float," which meant I may be on a different floor each night. Most of the floors have about the same routine, with minor variations.

I came to work at 11:00 p.m., checked with the patients, and was responsible for taking vital signs at midnight. From then on, unless someone needed something, I did not have to perform any duties until I took vital signs again at 4:00 a.m. The only other employee on that floor of the hospital was the nurse. When I refer to a floor, I mean a certain section of the hospital. For instance, the second floor actually consists of six sections: 2A (psychiatric), 2C (urology), 2D or 2E (medical), 2G (extended care), and 2F (orthopedic). Taking charge of each of these sections was a nurse, who usually had an aide to work with. When the patients slept—the hours between 1:00 a.m. and 4:00 a.m.—it could seem very long. Supper was served from 2:00 p.m. until 4:00 p.m., which gave a person something to do for at least half an hour. The other times provided excellent opportunities to get to know fellow employees if you wished, and each section of the floor was close enough to the next so that you could walk over and talk to the people working nearby and yet be close if you were needed on your own floor.

Other than obtaining information through participant observation, I also interviewed a nurse who works at the hospital. I chose Michele as an informant because she is a good friend of mine. The fact that I already had her trust, I thought, would make it easier for me to obtain the information. I have known her for about three years. The interview took place at her house during a Friday evening. I used a small tape recorder, which sat on the table in the living room while we sat on the couch and talked, sipping on cokes. The interview was quite informal, which made it easier to gather the information I was seeking. It only lasted about twenty minutes, but I was pleased with the responses I got to my questions. I had previously prepared a casual questionnaire to give me something to follow. The topics I covered dealt with questions about the morgue, hospital parties, the general atmosphere of working at night, stories told by fellow employees, and tricks played on other people working at the hospital. Other than the questionnaire, I just asked what came to mind while conducting the interview.

My informant's name is Michele DeGott. She is a registered nurse who is also a student at Western Kentucky University, working on her bachelor's degree. She is twenty-two years old, not married, and comes from Louisville. She now lives in Bowling Green and plans to stay here for at least another year and continue to work at the Bowling Green–Warren County Hospital. She then plans to continue her education in nursing and work toward her master's degree.

When I first began to work at the hospital, I noticed on certain nights there were dinner parties taking place on certain floors, and everyone seemed to be invited. These parties were usually for people's birthdays, or else they were going-away parties. The first time I noticed something unusual going on it was because I noticed that the cafeteria was virtually empty at dinner time and I wondered where everyone was and felt a little left out. I didn't know anybody well enough to ask what was going on. Michele said she wasn't invited to any parties at first either and said, "You knew about them but you didn't feel bad because you didn't know the people. It was like you had to prove yourself, then once you got in the group you were invited to all of them."

The way I first got invited is when someone came around to the floor with a sheet of paper to inform me who the party was being given for and asked me if I would come and bring something to eat, so I signed up. These dinners were usually given in a small room right off the nurses' station. All the food would be set up on the counters, and all who were invited would stop by during their thirty-minute dinner break and help themselves to an excellent meal. It would get quite crowded, and everyone would just stand up somewhere with their plates and talk to each other. Even the nurse supervisor would stop by for dinner. The food was always excellent. Often one person would be known for bringing a special dish which came to be his personal contribution. I remember that one nurse always brought chicken that was made with beer and everyone raved about how good it was, and it certainly was great. Somehow I felt that the party may not have been the same without her chicken.

These parties were always a happy affair. Most of them were supposed to have been surprise parties, but if a person had worked at the hospital for a long time it seemed as if they expected a party on their birthday. I enjoyed going because it provided an excellent opportunity to get to know new people. Once I had come to one party, I was invited to all of them. There were very few people that were not invited, especially if they had turned down an invitation and seemed to have no interest, or those people working on the labor and delivery floor.

As best I could understand, other hospital employees felt these people worked in a totally different world that was relatively stress free. I even noticed in the cafeteria that most of the obstetrics workers all ate together, or else they came down and got their food to take up to their floor with them. I worked on that floor and in the nursery several times and overheard stories one of the nurses had about their annual Christmas party. It seems as if they had their own party at one of the nurse's houses and didn't invite other hospital employees. Other than this one separate group, I found that night workers in the hospital tend to remain a closely knit bunch.

At night, when something goes wrong at the hospital chaos can easily break out. There just are not that many people there to handle a crisis on the floor, so the stress seems to be worse than it would be during the day. As Michele said,

> On nights you do all the work yourself. You don't have the facilities to just call the doctor. The doctors aren't as available. Six or seven doctors go in together, and you're not going to know if you're going to get the doctor that's in charge, or maybe the doctor on call, but that doctor may not know all the stuff about the patient. You have to decide if it's serious enough to call the doctor or is it not, since you are by yourself. It's like darkness doesn't give you the security that daylight does. When six o'clock comes around and the sun comes up, you feel good.

Another reason tension may be worse at night is because "there's no visitors, and most of the time when visitors are [not] there the patients are real serious. You get real caught up with the patients; you are depressed. Somehow things don't seem as bad during the day; there are more people to rely upon. At night you are the nurse; during days you've got two or three nurses on the floor."

One may think that if the tension is higher at night the workers would be more serious, but it seems to be just the opposite. Things on nights seem to be more informal, since there is an unwritten code among the nurses that no one wears their hats at night, like they do on the other shifts. As Michele points out, "Most of the people on nights are just friendlier and everybody is close. If you are having a bad time on a floor, everybody knows." It seems as if everyone shares their problems with the other workers. During dinner the discussion may center on what is going on on each person's floor and the problems that come up. These conversations seem to function as a release of tension during dinner, allowing people to return to their floors feeling better. I know that I always felt better about some of the bad things that happened if I could share it with another worker and hear that others were feeling the same way I did.

It is very common among day workers to think that at night the workers don't do anything. Michele says she hears this from day nurses many time[s]. Her feelings are that "some nights it is quiet; people sleep and you just walk around every hour to make sure they're all right." However, there is always a feeling of insecurity. "It's either quiet or it's crazy, and when it's quiet it's like you're waiting for something to happen."

During all this waiting many interesting things take place. People can think of all sorts of amusing diversions when times get quiet. One thing I noticed . . . that some employees enjoyed doing was taking a visit to the morgue. I admit that I was serious enough to go there just to see what it was like, but I would not want to go back just for pleasure. The morgue is down in the basement and no one works there at night, so it is dark and it seems so cold and impersonal. Anyone who was not busy could go down with the house orderly when he had to bring a body to the morgue. He had the keys and would sometimes just take people down if he wasn't busy. He also enjoyed scaring people and sometimes [would] make jokes about things like legs that may be found in his morgue refrigerator.

Another diversion, which is a bit more lighthearted than the last, was playing with the wheelchairs and stretchers left out in the halls. With a wheelchair you could have races by pushing people around in them and try to get them to fall out as you made sharp turns and fast stops, or you could try your skill at balancing on the back of one while someone steered from in the chair. There were games that could not be played if the nurse supervisor and certain other nurses were around, because they would frown upon such behavior.

Playing tricks on other employees is another way to pass time. One thing we used to do is call up and say strange things over the orderly's beeper. Certain workers would carry beepers with them, and to contact them you called a certain number on the telephone. A beeping noise was heard, and when it stopped you would tell them what you needed and then hang up. We often would call and give some weird message, then wait to see if the orderly could figure out who had called.

Another trick was to put stickers on workers' backs when they were not looking, so they would wear them around the hospital all night. There were many of these sticker tapes that said such things as "stool specimen," "strain urine," and "isolation." Scaring other employees was another trick that was often played. Other than the nurses' station, the floor is dark unless a patient happened to be up with a light on. When you made rounds you had to take a flashlight in order to see. It was easy, if you saw someone coming down the hall, to duck into a side room and jump out at them, scaring them to death.

Michele told me a story about a trick one of the nurse's aides played on the orderly one night. She said, "One of the aides went and got in the bed located in a room that was empty. Ralph [the orderly] knew this, since he checked the sheet before he went down there, because she [a patient] wanted some orange juice." Here I will explain that before taking a patient any food, one must check the diet sheet to see if it is permitted on their diet. The rooms have an intercom system in which the patient pushes a button and a light goes on in the nurses' station. The nurse can then push the lit button and talk to the patient over the intercom. This aide had disguised her voice to sound like an old lady and asked if she could please have some orange juice. The rest of Michele's story is as follows:

"Ralph said, 'There's nobody in that room.' The nurses said, 'Somebody just called for something. Obviously we've probably missed it, because we know she's down there. We've been checking on her all night.' Ralph goes down there, and she has the curtain drawn and is in the far bed. He pulls the curtain back, and she jumps out of bed. Ralph threw the orange juice all over her. The bed was soaked, and the juice was in her hair and all over her face. It was a riot; she scared the heck out of him!"

The patients also get bored and enjoy scaring workers to death when they enter the room at night. I've had several patients lie there quietly while I walked over to them very slowly so I could check them without disturbing their sleep. They would then wait until I was right next to them and say something or grab me. I never failed to jump, no matter how many times this trick had been played on me.

There was an elderly man in the hospital who had been there for a long time. Every night he was required to save his urine in a urinal beside his bed, which was collected each morning and taken to the lab. Well, he was a little senile and getting tired of all the routine, so he decided to stir up some commotion. What he did was sit up about an hour before someone usually came to collect his urine and go into the bathroom, dumping it out. He then filled it with apple juice and hung it by his bedside. When someone came to pick it up he grabbed it and drank the whole thing, which definitely stirred up the commotion he was looking for. This story may be a bit extreme, but it sure got the point across to me.

One lady I was taking care of on the psychiatric floor would pile up enormous wads of toilet tissues on her head and parade around the hall. One night I had to help her clean up, and I brought her a clean dressing gown to put on, and I left the room. A few minutes later she madly stormed out into the hall, naked, telling me I had given her a gown with a hole in it and she was too embarrassed to wear it!

Other stories are often told among employees, either when they are bored or during dinner time. The topics are varied, but one topic always heard among the night workers [is] lack-of-sleep stories. As Michele said, "That's the first comment relative to the three-to-eleven shift. Everybody complains they didn't sleep. It's never boring, since everyone can top everybody else. They give you ten thousand reasons why they didn't sleep." It's almost like a contest to see if you can beat another's story. The first thing I heard at the time clock each night was how much sleep everyone had, and I heard it again at dinner time. What amazed me were the workers who had worked this shift for ten years or more, and according to them, they never got any sleep!

It was difficult to sleep during the day sometimes, as I soon found out. People will invariably call or come over right after you've gone to bed. One day, while I tried to sleep through the construction that was going to next door and the heat in my apartment, the UPS man brought a package, a guy came to spray the apartment for roaches, my dog jumped on the bed and tried to put his pull toy in my hands at the time the phone rang, and when my neighbor across the hall began to hammer, I gave up and went to work tired. I told several stories that night just to keep myself awake. One thing that would infuriate me was when someone from the hospital would call during the time you were asleep and ask if you could please work extra time or for someone else. I would often turn them down just because I was mad.

There were always good stories to be heard about what other workers said when they answered the phone from a deep sleep—mostly harsh words. One nurse I knew told the hospital she would come in and work but took her phone off the hook, then went back to sleep and never remembered having been called. . . .

Telling stories, having parties, and other lighthearted attempts at having fun tend to ease the tension and make it easier to remain calm with the patients, even when things are going badly. I feel that without these interactions between worker[s] occurring, work may become unbearable and employees may tend to take home the tension instead of leaving it at the hospital when their shift is over.

Michele DeGott, Bowling Green, interviewed by Laurie Pennisi;
placed on deposit at Western Kentucky University Library,
Manuscripts and Archives, April 30, 1979

DEATH OF PRESIDENT KENNEDY

The only thing that stands out in my memory during the two years I spent living in Louisville and working in the hospitals and physicians' offices during the years 1962–1964 has nothing to do with patient care. Instead, it is the memory of that November 1963 afternoon I went to work. President John Fitzgerald Kennedy had just been assassinated.

I was pregnant, and the patients were concerned that I would worry too much and risk losing my baby. Every patient was listening to their radio in their room on the postpartum wing at the Kentucky Baptist Hospital. That was a sad day for all Americans.

Evelyn Pearl Anderson, July 18, 2012

INAPPROPRIATE RECOGNITION

At Pleasant Acres Nursing Home in Altamont, Illinois, we had a cute little lady named Allie Fry who was already past one hundred years of age. As a newly hired nurse I was pulling the midnight shift. All things seemed pretty quiet that night until suddenly Mrs. Allie appeared at the nurses' station, dressed in her Sunday best, hat and all.

When asked what she was doing, she replied, "I'm waiting for John to come and pick me up! He's supposed to be here in a minute!" We had a tough time convincing her that John would not be there that night and that she should go up to bed.

She repeated this process on several different nights. I was very curious about the whole thing so I decided to try to find out who John was. I supposed he had been her husband but was amazed to find he had actually been her father!

Charlene Vaught, Portland, TN, August 2, 2011

CARING FOR OBESE PATIENTS

This story is about a morbidly obese woman I met [along] with a home health nurse. Our assignment was to change the dressing on her sacral wound. The only warning I got was that this patient was bedridden and rather large. I had never imagined that a person could become so obese that this could cause them to become bedridden. This lady entirely filled a king-sized bed and was sitting squarely in the middle of the bed, watching TV and eating a burger. Since that time I have met many patients struggling with their addiction to food.

Obesity in America is a complete epidemic. It is so sad to see a human completely break down and just watch the self-remorse that they have for the destruction they have waged on their own bodies. They cannot walk without getting out of breath, and some have been instructed by an orthopedic doctor that they risk fracturing their legs if they try to bear their own weight. They cannot perform basic tasks and are reduced to asking a family member to assist them while toileting. They are instantly judged by the world the very second they step out of the comfort of their homes. The crux of their pain is that they did it to themselves and they feel too far gone to do anything about it, so they eat more to cope with how they are feeling.

Louise Webb, Bowling Green, June 10, 2013

10

GOVERNMENTAL AND BUSINESS ISSUES

Stories in this chapter relate the role of the federal government in health care and business concerns of medical institutions. Some reveal how much the Frontier Nursing Service and its staff members, as well as local doctors and area residents, needed financial support. These stories also bring into focus the slowness of payments from Medicaid and Medicare and describe the receipt of food stamps. Many, many local residents, especially students, used to live without adequate food supplies, water, and adequate heating. The Frontier Nursing Service was often out of reach for some backcountry families. However, the FNS did take boxes of food and clothing to those they knew about and could reach.

The federal government did so very much for these mountain people, but sometimes it was still not enough. Thankfully, the government did build a number of rather primitive houses for families truly in need. Also, during the Great Depression the federal government employed a lot of local men to work for the Works Projects Administration (WPA) and the Civilian Conservation Corps (CCC).

MEDICAID AND MEDICARE

I came to the Frontier Nursing Service in October 1965. Before that I had been a Sister of Charity and had been in India for six years. I came back in 1964 for reasons of health and left the order in 1965 and began trying to find a place that needed my particular set of talents. Frontier Nursing was recommended by a physician in Louisville, as they were looking for somebody very desperately at that particular time. I went on down there several months before I left the order. I was familiar with that part of Kentucky only by hearsay. I did have a pretty good idea as to what it would be like, since I had worked in relatively backward rural areas. I assumed it would be like what I was familiar with while in India.

Dr. W. B. Rogers (or Beasley?) was getting ready to go to England for a DPH, DTH, or DTM, just whatever it was [doctor of public health degree, DrPH], and as he was leaving just about that time and they were interested in getting somebody to keep up the continuity. So I got there just shortly after he left and began working in the old hospital. The Frontier Nursing Service medical staff members filled out the needed forms and got things taken care of, and I signed them all by the thousands. Medicare was always behind [in] its payments to us. I remember one year I was there that Medicare sent us word that they had overpaid us $900 the previous year, and we hadn't been paid by them for three years or something like that. What they overpaid us we'd never seen, because they were so far behind in their payments. So I know we were doing it, and I know I signed innumerable Medicaid, Medicare papers.

Told by Dr. Mary Wiss to Dale Deaton, February 14, 1979;
provided by the Louie B. Nunn Center for Oral History,
University of Kentucky Libraries, Lexington

GOVERNMENT MONEY

The Frontier Nursing Service is unique in that it's in a rural setting and it is isolated, and for someone like me who's going to another rural setting in Nicaragua that is isolated, this is a good place to come to see how I, as a person, react to that, not only to the isolation but also to the independence that isolation gives you. They allow us to use our skills quite independently, not only in the clinics, but you also have to provide for yourself recreation, an hour's rest and relaxation.

I think the FNS prepares people for rural settings, and that's why I chose FNS in the first place. Now that I'm leaving, I really feel it has been a good experience in that regard.

With a lot of government involvement in health, nursing, and medical care, I think poor people are well cared for, and I don't think anymore that we need to give large sums of [government] money just to take care of the poor. I think we need to give money to take care of the middle class, and because the third-party payments are paying the cost of everything. The reason why the cost has gone up is because we know we can collect a certain amount from the government. But we have to be uniform across the board, and so everybody ends up paying the same price. I think it's the lower-middle-class people who are out working and do not qualify for help. I think they're the ones caught in the crunch, and I think they are the ones not receiving health care because they're not able to pay for it. I don't know how you could give money to that class of people, because they're the strong type of people who have pride and they're out wanting to make their own way. But I've had a lot of concern about that, and the Frontier Nursing Service is starting to be out of reach for some of these people.

Told by Karen Slabaugh to Dale Deaton, March 23, 1979;
provided by the Louie B. Nunn Center for Oral History,
University of Kentucky Libraries, Lexington

GOVERNMENT SUPPORT

In the midsixties along came VISTA and the War on Poverty, such things as food stamps, Medicare, Medicaid, and other things. I think that when those programs came in, especially the school lunch program, which was more meaningful than any of the others, [they] made a difference in the hemoglobins and the blood of the schoolchildren. They weren't as anemic. In fact, you could tell a big difference in the preschoolers and the schoolchildren because of the school lunch program. They were getting a balanced diet and getting good. . . . And when the food stamp program came, people could buy what they wanted. I always got upset over the fact that people could buy a lot of pop and junk food rather than buying the things that I felt like they needed. At that time you couldn't buy soap, and I thought what a silly thing it was that they couldn't buy soap because it was a much-needed commodity. . . .

I can't remember whether it was Peace Corps or VISTA, but they had these young folks assigned to Lost Fork, which had a very bad road on its way up the mountain. You had to cross several creeks [and] thus truly needed a jeep to get up there. I remember that these [young] folks were living up there and they rented themselves a modern, up-to-date car from Avis Rent-A-Car, but there was no way that that car could get up and down. Well, they just tore it up, but our tax money was going to rent that car every day for those folks. It was just not well done at all.

The [government] wanted to build outhouses for the people, since many of them didn't have any kind of indoor plumbing or outdoor plumbing at all. They just used the back of the house [as a toilet]. So instead of soliciting people's cooperation or building it with them, [the government] built it for them. They wanted to use natural things that were available, so they put up this makeshift thing, using the hood of the car located on the front of the outhouse. But the back was just as open as can be, and there was this huge, huge hole that children could have fallen into. Actually, it was never built and was not even a sanitary privy. Of course, the people wouldn't use it, but the workers thought they were really doing something. So I didn't think that was so great! But as far as some of these other federal programs, there's much more money than has become available to the people.

As the years went by I had to look hard to find families that were really destitute or really in need of help. When I first came there were dozens of families for which we could fix food boxes and clothes boxes. When I left the Red Bird District in 1970 I could count on just one hand the families that needed help, and mainly that was because the husband was recently out of work, someone had died in the family, or something like that. At that point in time most people had much more available to them.

Told by Elsie Maier to Dale Deaton, December 5, 1978;
provided by the Louie B. Nunn Center for Oral History,
University of Kentucky Libraries, Lexington

FEDERAL HELPFULNESS

To continue my story about the federal government, let me say that the feds helped with housing also. As long as you did the work, they would supply the materials. So a lot of people put siding on their homes and renovated them and did a lot to get their homes in better condition. That was really a marked improvement. Another big trend that happened through the years was the moving of the people down from the hollows to the main road. And some of this was done on their own efforts, because of getting their children to school and being available for work and things of that sort. But part of it also was due to the enforcement of the rules for the Daniel Boone National Forest and the Red Bird National Forest area. And when the federal government bought all that land that was previously owned by Red Bird Timber Corporation and Fordson Company, a lot of people were living on that property and paying very little, if any at all, for the house they were in. They weren't forced out of their homes, but they were told that as soon as the main provider of the house died they would have to move. And they were not allowed to raise tobacco or any money crop, but they could raise enough corn to feed their own stock. They had to keep their livestock within fences. All these rules forced them off the property, because they couldn't survive up in the hollows without having a big garden. Since many of them lived off the land, that order created a lot of resentment and hard feelings.

In fact, there was a Smokey the Bear sign put up right by the forestry located at the Double Creek turnoff, and that sign was shot down so many times the [government officials] finally decided they would leave him [Smokey] down. The federal government was kind of angry over it, but I think the federal programs really have helped to give people more money.

Told by Elsie Maier to Dale Deaton, December 5, 1978;
provided by the Louie B. Nunn Center for Oral History,
University of Kentucky Libraries, Lexington

FEDERAL GOVERNMENT SUPPORT

Before I went to Hyden in 1938 I knew so little about Mrs. Breckinridge and the Frontier Nursing Service. I actually went down there rather ignorant of the whole thing, but I really liked the idea because I was an eager horsewoman and loved the idea of doing something useful that was connected with horses. While I was there I went on several baby deliveries at their homes. Sometimes I even entertained the rest of the family, especially the little children.

It was said that back then a lot of assistance was given out by the federal government, and a lot of men worked on the WPA and the CCC. It was also said that the FNS had clothes, food, canned milk, and formulas for babies that they gave out.

Told by Martha Webster, Appletree, OH, to Dale Deaton,
March 4, 1979; provided by the Louie B. Nunn Center
for Oral History, University of Kentucky Libraries, Lexington

SANITARY TOILETS NEEDED

I was in the judge's office when people were worried because they thought the waters of Buck Horn Lake were being contaminated, and that wasn't too long ago. I was in Judge Wooten's office and heard this man say, "Well, Judge, the best thing to do is put them in jail if they don't build sanitary toilets."

I burst out laughing, and Judge Wooten heard me and then introduced me to this federal guy that was there, who said to me, "I hear you laughing."

I said, "Yes, I'm amused. . . . I couldn't help hearing that you're gonna put a man in jail because he didn't have a sanitary toilet, so I want to know who's gonna dig? If he's behind bars, then no one can dig. What he needs is a little bit in the supplies, and you have plans in the health department where they always had good plans for sanitary toilets."

Kinda stunned, he said, "You're right."

My response was, "I know I am right, and if you put him behind bars, he can't build his toilet. You can't help people unless you understand how they're thinking."

This is true of the world, isn't it?

Told by Helen E. Browne, Wendover, to Dale Deaton, March 27, 1979;
provided by the Louie B. Nunn Center for Oral History,
University of Kentucky Libraries, Lexington

BAD SITUATIONS FOR SOME ELDERLY PERSONS

Before [the term] Alzheimer's [came into use], this condition in older individuals was called organic brain syndrome, or dementia, with the cause attributed to hardening of the arteries. Alzheimer's was known more as a condition that afflicted a younger population, those in their early fifties. Irregardless of the cause of the dementia, many were institutionalized as late as the 1970s. You didn't see people with severe mental health issues, as they were in institutions.

There was a shift to placing individuals with mental health conditions into community settings. They live independently or with families that can monitor them. Unfortunately many are not able to manage on their own. Many in the homeless population are individuals with psychiatric disorders, living on riverbanks and [in] abandoned buildings. A growing number of these are men and women who have served in the military.

While institutions were not ideal institutions and we should not go back to those conditions, we must find some better way to take care of those who cannot take care of themselves and require some type of custodial care.

Patricia A. Slater, Petersburg, March 6, 2013

11

Medications in Earlier Times

This chapter includes insightful information about medications used during pioneer times as well as during the early to mid-1900s. Nurse-midwives, and in earlier times even some untrained servants, provided services and medications to numerous patients. Some women were given such a variety of pills that they had to provide detailed diary descriptions of any other forms of medication that they might be taking, such as natural herbs, vinegar, and numerous homegrown items, including sassafras tea. I personally remember, during my growing-up years in Monroe County, a husband and wife who had never been to see a doctor, but both lived to their early nineties. They both drank tea made from natural sources and daily took a variety of natural herbs.

Included in these stories is praise for midwives who did baby deliveries and pioneer doctors who transported their medications in saddlebags. Some of their helpful items included things made with knives and paper bags.

Healthy Old Couple

I remember one old couple that lived not far from my center on Beach Fork, and I used to ride over that [there], which was the place you could go six miles on a horse or thirty miles in the jeep. Needless to say, I usually took the horse. There were several families in the area, and I could sort of make a round-robin that way. This old couple lived in a house that I think had one room, and I know it had zero windows, and the door stood open during the summer and even in winter to let some light in. The wife cooked on a fireplace grate because they had no stove.

She made the best biscuits from the top of the flour sack, absolutely delicious. I am not a stickler about cleanliness, so I always ate her biscuits, even though her fingers were black with coal [dust]. I figured coal was probably very healthy and never worried about it. If it were anywhere close to mealtime she always had a biscuit with jelly on it for me.

I always took the man's blood pressure and bawled him out about the grease. He was the one that would go and dig the sing [ginseng], and he'd be better the next time I came by, but by the third time I came he'd run out of sing and his blood pressure was back up again.

As far as I know they both lived to a ripe old age. They were very friendly old people, and I remember them very clearly.

Told by Jean Fee to Rebecca Adkins Fletcher, June 15, 2002;
provided by the Louie B. Nunn Center for Oral History,
University of Kentucky Libraries, Lexington

EARLY BIRTH CONTROL PILLS

An interesting thing we were doing in Leslie County in 1958 was peddling birth control pills, although other places were not doing this. The reason we were doing that is because we were a field-testing site for Dr. John [Rock]'s pill that he had just invented. It was first invented as fertility treatment. Then the realization was, "Hey, we're stopping ovulation in these people to see if, when we withdraw the medications, they'll actually ovulate, and thereby get pregnant; which [what] else can we do by stopping ovulation?" So we were doing field trial[s] for the honorable Dr. John, and he came and lectured to us as a class. What made me think about that was that I received that lecture while reclining on a couch, courtesy of the penicillin shots that I was also receiving at the time.

We were doing field trials, and therefore contraceptive pills were available to the women of our service area long before they were available to the general public. Wasn't that a blessing! There were quite a number of them who, for reasons of their own feelings on the subject or for reasons of their husband's feeling on the subject, didn't participate in those trials. And they weren't controlled trials, where you gave some sugar pills to some women and the real thing to others. That would have been totally unethical, but we did require each woman to keep a very detailed diary and to bring it with her every month to the clinic. But if no diary, then no more pills.

We nurses would make sure we mentioned it when there was nobody else in earshot, typically at the clinic, because there were a lot of people who had, and a few who still had, strong beliefs against birth control pills of any kind.

Told by Jean Fee to Rebecca Adkins Fletcher, June 15, 2002;
provided by the Louie B. Nunn Center for Oral History,
University of Kentucky Libraries, Lexington

HOME REMEDIES

Some people were very good preparing and using home remedies made with local herbs. I think of one old lady who had a complete dresser with all the drawers full of various herbs stuck down in little bags and jars. They were either labeled or not labeled, but she professed to know what they all were and what to do with each one. Maybe she did. She was a relative of Phil, who had a lesser opinion of them. But there were some particularly old women that knew a lot about herbs and would use them. I really don't know how effective they were.

People would put vinegar and brown paper on a sprain, and it worked as well as anything else does for a sprain. Time is what a sprain takes, and being off it. And the vinegar and brown paper probably did make it feel better. They knew how to make [poultices], and so did my mother. Remember, we didn't have easy access to antibiotics, so if you got an infection all you had to do, according to them, was draw the poison out.

We had some beliefs that seemed peculiar to me, and there are still all kinds of people that think getting your head wet gives you a cold. In my books, a virus gives you a cold, but there are still lots of people that think getting your head wet, or getting some other part of you wet, gives you a cold. . . . They used sassafras tea for a number of different things, partly because it tastes pretty good and it was supposed to make a number of things better.

I have to admit being a lot less appreciative of home remedies at that time in my life. And as you know, herbs and various alternative things are much more popular now than they were around ten years ago. There's a resurgence in using them these days. When you stop to think about it, where did all of our pills and potions that we prescribe come from? They all came from nature somewhere. Some of them are synthesized in the lab, and those that are synthesized occurred in nature. Some of them we use come straight from nature, like Premarin and digitalis, and we put them in a packet and put a label on them and call them pharmaceuticals.

Told by Jean Fee to Rebecca Adkins Fletcher, June 15, 2002;
provided by the Louie B. Nunn Center for Oral History,
University of Kentucky Libraries, Lexington

MIDWIVES' BABY DELIVERIES

In doing normal midwifery, I think a midwife has far better training than a physician has. Midwives know how to manage a woman to relax her so that she can have a more normal birth. And they stay with her afterwards to help her care for herself and her baby. Midwives don't just deliver the baby and then walk out of the room, they stay with her and support her. They also help to create the bond between the mother and her baby, which is quite different than what medicine does.

I'm not against what medicine does if it is needed. . . . I just reviewed a study of obstetrics that was done in this country during the early 1960s relative to sixteen thousand deliveries. That was the last extensive study done in this country, and it was appalling how much medical care was considered routine. I truly think the mother is much better off if she is delivered normally.

Told by Gertrude Isaacs to Dale Deaton, November 15, 1978;
provided by the Louie B. Nunn Center for Oral History,
University of Kentucky Libraries, Lexington

LACK OF MONEY FOR MEDICATIONS

I think nurses suffered from not knowing enough about local things. We probably didn't have enough orientation as how to use them. If we wanted to get something done, the barn man was on the committee, and he would help us committee members by doing things for us.

Looking now at money availability, back in those days we were supposed to collect two dollars a year from the families, which meant they were covered for the nurses' care in the home for that small amount of money. And it was really hard to collect that two dollars from many, many people because they didn't have it to spare. A lot of bartering took place, and bartering means someone would bring a sack of corn to pay for something else. They also would swap pigs, etc.

I didn't come into the hospital until 1958, and then in 1959 or 1960 a lady paid her whole maternity bill and [for] her cholecystectomy that she had afterwards in eggs for two and one-half years. She paid me in eggs, and I bought the eggs and gave her money for petty cash that we did have from the service. We put the cost onto her bill, sent it to her, and she eventually paid that bill. It took her thirty months to pay that bill, but that's just an example of how proud some people were and how they would work out their bill.

Told by Molly Lee to Carol Crowe-Carraco, February 6, 1979;
provided by the Louie B. Nunn Center for Oral History,
University of Kentucky Libraries, Lexington

EARLY HEALING PRACTICES

My grandmother was the first public health nurse that I ever knew of in Leslie County. She was not a midwife, nor was she a granny woman. That was my father's mother, Peggy Lewis, and their home was right there where John Lewis's house is now, the big stone house. There was a big log house there at one time, with a wide hall in the middle and rooms on each side and in the back, and upstairs. It was a beautiful old log house and I can remember it. The Presbyterian Church bought it and built the dormitory which later was acquired by John Lewis.

As I understand it, Grandmother had methods of taking care of the sick that are still good today. I don't know how it ever came into my hands, but upstairs we have her doctor book, a big dictionary type, a big, thick book. My husband gets the biggest pleasure out of reading in it about the remedies they used back then. Wherever there was sickness, my grandmother was called. She was just a housekeeper in the community, but she had a knack for taking care of the sick. So wherever there was sickness of any kind she was called to come. She took care of sick babies, and of course, back then dysentery and diarrhea were the plague of the country, caused by polluted water and everything like that. Some people even had bloody flux every summer, which is a severe form of diarrhea and dysentery. But Grandmother had remedies which are good even today.

A personal note about my father's brother, Sam Lewis, who was the third child in the family and who eventually went to medical school. That was the joy of his mother's life. She couldn't wait until Sam got through medical school in Louisville, where my father went to law school, and come back home to doctor the sick, because there was no trained doctor here at that time.

As I said, Mama was a nurse and went around taking care of the sick, who had typhoid and everything like that. Just about the time John graduated from medical school he died of tuberculosis. He left a young widow, who was a beautiful, devoted woman, and their little child. Their child was frail and died from tuberculosis. They called it galloping consumption back then. . . . Then this Aunt Mary, about whom I have spoken of so affectionately, died of tuberculosis. It is sad to see all of their graves there behind the Presbyterian church.

Of course, Grandmother had this great disappointment because she had looked forward to this doctor coming into the community. It's very interesting to me to have heard about all the things she did as a nurse. Mother always said that Grandmother practiced methods in nursing service that were good and were acceptable even today. And reading in her book, it makes good sense that she used the remedies that she used.

Told by Mary Lewis Biggerstaff, Berea, to Dale Deaton,
February 13, 1979; provided by the Louie B. Nunn Center
for Oral History, University of Kentucky Libraries, Lexington

PIONEER DOCTORS

There were a couple of primitive doctors in Hyden during the 1910s and so forth. They were Dr. [Jack?] Huff and Dr. Lewis. I want to emphasize that I think Dr. John Lewis served a great mission there and relieved illness a great deal with the limited information that he had. Dr. Jack is so proud of him. Jack got his medical pockets that he carried on this little horse. Then there was a young Dr. Joe Lawrence who also came in there. He was from Mt. Vernon, where he had married a beautiful girl, Tana Morgan. In Leslie County they lived at Short Creek in an old house I still remember. Dr. Joe delivered me when I was born in 1899. Dr. Joe died, and his brother Dr. George Lawrence came there and practiced medicine for quite a while.

Back then the doctors could give pills and calomel [for intestinal worms] and other things like that. I remember calomel [was quite effective]. The doctor would put a little bit of calomel [powder] on the point of a knife and then wrap it in paper. I don't remember what else doctors used back then, but we never had to take much medicine.

There was a Dr. Edward Ray and his brother, Dr. Robert Ray, that came in from West Virginia and set up a drugstore in Hyden during the early 1900s, across the street from the courthouse. Dr. Bob Ray had a son, Lyle Ray, who is a druggist here in Berea now. These two doctor brothers were upstanding citizens, and they made a great contribution to Leslie County. Dr. [name not specified] Ray had a son, Manuel, who became a doctor and worked with the Veterans Administration in Lexington.

After the railroad came to Hazard, Dr. Ray went over there as a company doctor and really worked himself to death serving the needs of the people there. There was also a Dr. Collins in Hazard who was a surgeon. He used to come to Hyden and helped with the Frontier Nursing Service.

Told by Mary Lewis Biggerstaff, Berea, to Dale Deaton,
February 12, 1979; provided by the Louie B. Nunn Center
for Oral History, University of Kentucky Libraries, Lexington

FOLK MEDICATIONS

While working at Frontier Nursing Service I didn't see any local medical practices that conflicted with regular medicine, but there were a lot of midwives' tales that focused on natural things they believed in at the time. When Mary Breckinridge started the Frontier Nursing Service in 1925, the women in the mountains of eastern Kentucky were tended to by lay midwives who had no health education, but they just helped out when they got a call from someone saying, "My wife's having her baby."

The mountain people back then had such myths as putting an axe under the bed to cut the pain and believing that an unborn baby could be strangled by the umbilical cord if the mother lifted her arms above her head.

Even at that time (1964) I was there when babies were born, and we would put what was called a belly band around them to keep the umbilical site from bulging out or maybe herniating. We know now that it wasn't necessary to do all that.

Told by Martha Hill, Glendale, to Mark Brown, June 30, 2012;
provided by the Kentucky Historical Society, Frankfort

DEATH

I recall the elderly woman who died just after I had given her morning medications. I was so stunned at how quickly life left and death came, or was it together? I was glad I had wrapped a shawl around her in the early morning hours so she would be warm.

It was always a humbling experience to close the eyes of a patient for the final time, knowing that the soul within was already gone from earth and that you were present to witness the event this side of heaven.

Evelyn Pearl Anderson, London, July 18, 2012

FOLK HEALING ITEMS

I recall cancer patients wanting their pinto beans from home and their water from their well. There was one refrigerator on the floor or area where the patient was situated. It was full of jars of cooked beans and water with the specific patient's name. I do not know that science has ever proved or even looked at a study on the relationship of pinto beans and personal water's effect on the quality of life.

I recall many farmers having to sell their farms in order to pay for some family member's hospital stay. In the days before Medicare and Medicaid came along there was indigent care, but no one really wanted to be placed in the category.

Those are things I'll never forget.

Evelyn Pearl Anderson, London, July 18, 2012

DEADLY INSECTICIDES

We nurses did all the x-rays at the hospital in Missouri. The temperature of solution to process the x-rays was dependent on the temperature outside. We learned to test the temperature of the solution with our fingers in order to estimate the time required for processing. It was very exciting to develop a "perfect" x-ray.

One day a patient was admitted. He was a farmer who had been using some new pesticides on his fields. The wind was blowing strongly, resulting in the farmer breathing an excessive amount of the dust. He wore no mask, as no need was known to do so. I took a large x-ray, as directed. Thus, a perfect x-ray was developed, revealing large holes in the various lobes of his lungs that were caused by damage from the insecticide. The patient died later on that same day.

I suspect that these types of cases started the requirement for labeling hazard cautions on products.

Evelyn Pearl Anderson, London, July 18, 2012

RATIONALE FOR VARIOUS MEDICATIONS

A squire or a magistrate from a local district came to the meeting of fiscal court in Hyden and became very ill at the Blue Wing Hotel and sent for the nurse at the girls' dormitory and asked her to come see him. The squire's two sons were sent because they were too embarrassed to call for the nurse. They went back and told their father that the nurse wouldn't come. Well, that irritated the squire, so he sent word to the other members of the fiscal court to take that [nurse's payment] off the book, since they were not to pay the twenty-five-dollar cost.

The cashier of the bank heard about this and came to the dormitory to ask if I knew about this man being sick, and I said no. Then the cashier asked if the sons had come after me. I said, "No, I never saw them." Then he asked if I would go now, and I said, "Yes."

I went and found a very sick man, and Dr. Collins had already been called from Hazard. I waited for Dr. Collins, and before he left he asked me if I would spend the night, because he didn't think it wise to let any other [person] give the medication that he was leaving for the sick man, so I agreed to stay that night. Well, in the morning the sick man was feeling a little better, and I knew I had to get back to do the other things I had to do, so I said to him, "I'll just give you a bath and things, then I'm gonna leave you."

So I called for clean sheets and we fixed him and everything up.

The only thing I found when I changed the linen [was that I] ran my hand into a cold steel pistol, so I asked his wife if she would come and remove the pistol, and she did. So after I left, the man changed his mind and told the fiscal court to put my name back on the book [for payment]. In the meantime, John Asher heard about this and called me and called the fiscal court together. He wanted me to hear what he had to say, and so I did. After his lecture, my only response was that if they didn't want to have the nurse, I didn't have to stay, and that would be perfectly all right. . . .

But after the close of the session I met Miss Zilpha Roberts . . . , and we became friends and she told me she would help find a place for me to live in Leslie County. The squire from the Cutshin District immediately said, "Well, I'll find a place for you to live if you'll start serving the schools."

I agreed, and they assigned me to five schools, where many children had the trachoma [virus]. After some time, I took seven or nine children to Jackson, where there was a state clinic.

Told by Jean Tolk, Barbourville, to Dale Deaton, November 1, 1978; provided by the Louie B. Nunn Center for Oral History, University of Kentucky Libraries, Lexington

INTRODUCING TYPHOID FEVER SHOTS

There was typhoid fever and other ailments in Dryhill, Leslie County, and people had not been vaccinated, just as it was in Buckhorn while I was there. I found a man in Dryhill who had typhoid. I began to inquire and found out that nobody had ever given typhoid shots to local residents, so when I started with the students they were all scared to death and wanted to run home. Mr. Murdock said to them, "If you do that the school will break up, and everything." It was really a problem, because it needed to be done.

The man in Dryhill [thought he] was dying with typhoid and living right on a little stream into which everything was poured out. However, he changed his mind later on. At Dryhill and Hyden I did the same thing but had nowhere to do my vaccinations except in our living room in the cottage.

I also remember a great big six-foot man kneeling over at church to pray because he was too scared to take a shot for typhoid.

Nobody had ever had typhoid before and nobody had ever been vaccinated.

Told by Jean Tolk, Barbourville, to Dale Deaton, November 1, 1978;
provided by the Louie B. Nunn Center for Oral History,
University of Kentucky Libraries, Lexington

MEDICATION ERRORS

Making a medication error is unforgettable and often [is] not much discussed among nurses. We hate for it to happen and live in fear of it happening. We have smart, computerized systems and try to prevent this from happening, but yet it does happen. I know the mistakes I have made by giving medication [via] the wrong route. It should have been an intramuscular injection but I gave it in the IV. As soon as I finished doing it I realized with dread what I had done.

What is the best thing to do in this situation? And the answer is to own up as soon as you can. So you apologize to the patient, monitor them closely for side effects, call the doctor, tell your manager, and then fill out an incident report, and you completely hate yourself. What you can do once it is done is learn from it and share with others to prevent it happening again.

Why do medication errors happen, since they can be deadly and literally cost lives? There are just a multitude of possible reasons why, since it is ultimately human and mistakes happen. On average, nurse-patient ratios are 6:1. However, what needs to be considered is the acuity of how sick each patient is, and these days the acuity of how sick a patient is on a regular med-surg floor is ever increasing. It is not an uncommon scenario for a nurse to be giving a blood transfusion to one patient and be needing to give pain medication and routine medications to other patients. Then change someone's dressing, then go fix someone's IV pump because air is in the line. Then your lovely Alzheimer patient decides she needs to go home and starts walking off down the hallway.

The doctor is on the phone wanting to give you an order, and of course, you have a new admission coming and they need to give you report about this patient right now. So when you throw all these situations together, the abilities that a nurse needs to stay levelheaded and be able to multitask and prioritize and not [to] make a medication error are complex.

Louise Webb, Bowling Green, June 10, 2013

Little Red Wagon

I suppose I could be called a pioneer, riding a wagon toward the northeast when only thirteen months and twelve days old. It was a time past the threat of Indians attacking those on the rural frontier. This particular "frontier" was divided by barbed wire fences running parallel to any old wagon road connecting two paved roadways, one of which was the Maysville Road. Beyond the fence on [the] left side of this old wagon road was the Vanlandingham farm. My father was hired to help on this farm, where a small house was located.

Moving to this house represented independence for my parents, as they had lived with their parents during the first two years of their marriage. In late 1938 I was born in a small farmhouse located about a half mile back off the Maysville Road on the left of the old wagon road. Dr. Graham came to the farmhouse, located about three miles out of Flemingsburg, to deliver me early one Tuesday morning. A lady had come to stay with Mother following my birth to help Mother and me for a month. This was part of rural health back in that decade [and] into the next. Women weren't supposed to do anything for about six weeks in order for the then-believed healing to take place.

My father made the giant decision to become a tenant farmer for

Mr. McCartney, who was county attorney. This sixty-some-acres farm in Fleming County was located on the other side of the old wagon road, separated by a barbed wire fence on the right. Then, on January 19, 1940, my parents moved into a large pre–Civil War house. It must have seemed like a mansion compared to the four-room house where they had lived. It was a cold mansion but very spacious, heated with coal stoves in two rooms.

My mother wrote in her five-year diary on this January 19, 1940, day the following account: "We moved to the McCartney place Friday when the temperature was around fourteen below zero, snow on." Both of my parents told me of my father pulling me through the snowy fields in a little red wagon to get to our new farmhouse.

One can only imagine how bundled up I must have been. According to my mother's diary, I had begun walking two days earlier. On January 22, 1940, she wrote, "Court Day, we went to town in afternoon and then put up our new mail box." Thus the story of farm life beginning for me was a taste of rural health, before my knowledge. That was my home until leaving for nurse's school in 1957.

In June 1944 my brother was born at home. The family doctor who was a general practitioner came to the house for the delivery. Actually, it was the same doctor that had delivered me at the small house. Jude was the lady who was hired to care for mother's postdelivery and to be the family housekeeper for at least a month. I recall wanting to go into the living room's delivery area when I heard the baby cry, but Jude would not let me go in. She very calmly kept on plaiting my hair in two braids, and I was okay.

The next time that I recall rural health being given in our home was about four years later, when I came down with a "serious case" of scarlet fever. The county public health doctor came to the house to check the report of scarlet fever. As he was leaving, I can hear in my mind's ears the thump, thump, thump of a hammer beating nails into the door. He had hung a bright "Quarantine—Scarlet Fever" sign on the front door. I had to remain quietly in the house for a month. Thankfully, no one else in the family became ill with this disease. Soon thereafter people received their shots at the doctor's office or in the local hospital, as the physician deemed necessary.

Fast forward to 1993, when I had been a registered nurse for many years and my last position had been as an executive director of a hospital. I had resigned that position due to a move resulting to my husband's change of employment. One day I received a telephone call from a nearby hospital inviting me to interview for the position of manager to their existing rural health clinic (RHC). This RHC was already licensed, certified, and located on the hospital campus. Before that, I was offered the position that sounded very interesting and challenging, so I accepted. I would learn on the job about RHCs.

During the following months I learned all I could about the Medicare/Medicaid licensed and certified rural health clinics. There are two types, which are freestanding or hospital based. They existed for medically underserved people located within nonurbanized area[s] as defined by the U.S. Census Bureau, and as in our case, [had to] be located in a medically underserved area under Section 330(b)(3) of the Public Health Service Act. These clinics were required to do some blood tests on site: urinalysis, hemoglobin, hematocrit, blood sugar, pregnancy tests, and primary culturing, for transmittal to a certified laboratory.

At that time only nurse-midwives were on the staff of the existing RHC. We added an internist and a pediatrician to the staff. This required a renovation of the existing building and the addition of new staff members, composed of a LPN [licensed practical nurse] and aide, plus receptionists for each of the two new physicians. Renovations are never easy, but all in all there was staff cooperation in this process as I began conferring with others related to their ideas. Pediatrics proved to be a needed service for the area. That practice grew the most rapidly. An obstetrician was added to the existing obstetrical/gynecological service being offered by the certified nurse-midwives.

As a registered nurse, I was concerned about the quality of patient care being offered. Ongoing performance-improvement studies were being held. A new concern and learning process for me, other than the renovation, was the coding and billing processes. These are essential in order to receive maximum reimbursement from Medicare and Medicaid. These monies were necessary in order to provide the services needed.

During my employment with this southeast Kentucky hospital my title changed to clinical outreach manager, and two more rural health clinics were added under this hospital umbrella. One was in a neighboring county, where we negotiated and purchased a building being used as a community restaurant. It is always difficult to take away a community restaurant that serves as a meeting place or a break room within a facility. People like the place where they eat!

I must say that the negotiations, renovations, and operations were fascinatingly pleasing. The hospital CEO was a skillful administrator who remained supportive throughout these processes. Once this newly renovated RHC had been licensed and certified by the Kentucky Licensure and Regulation [Department] we were able to open the doors following a community open house. This RHC offered medical care and obstetrical care by two nurse practitioners. The obstetrician at the first rural health clinic would drive the thirty-some miles once a week to see patients and to serve as a backup to the certified nurse-midwife. The hospital had a rural health clinic contract with the dentist in the county seat to receive referrals from this second clinic. The dental service was very important to offer this community, as uninsured persons needing dental care would be able to have the necessary care rendered. The dentist would submit a bill to the hospital with reimbursement through the RHC Medicare/Medicaid billing process. I have never known if we broke even, but I do know that for a couple of patients the dental work given was life changing.

In the next few months we opened a third RHC, which was located about twenty miles east of the hospital and the first clinic. This clinic was housed in a renovated mobile office unit. The very capable maintenance staff members at the hospital were wonderful to work with throughout all of these renovations. This clinic also had to go through the inspection process for Medicare/Medicaid licensure by the Kentucky Licensure and Regulation.

The third clinic was supervised by and patient care was given by an older, experienced nurse practitioner. Mary [Breckinridge] ran a top-notch RHC. Her staff had to be employed to assist in the overall operations of this clinic, as [they] had been for the other two.

During the first three years the staff suffered some tragedy. One of the LPNs of the first clinic was killed in an automobile accident one evening after work. Later, the husband of one of the LPNs was killed when the bulldozer he was driving rolled over [on] a hillside, pinning him beneath. The small village community came quickly to the aid of the LPN and her family. Many of those [who suffered tragedy] were patients of the third RHC. Such tragedies have an emotional effect on the employees and members of the small communities.

Although I did not function in a traditional registered nurse capacity, I did do interviews and studies to ensure that quality health care was being given at each end of the clinics. Each rural health clinic was to do annual program evaluation and to be recertified for licensure and certification every year. We worked as a team to ensure the standards were being met.

The RHCs of today differ from my Fleming County, Kentucky,

"rural health" of yesteryear. However, the goal of healing care remained the same. It was even possible that a daddy could pull his child in a little red wagon to any one of our three clinics.

Evelyn Pearl Anderson, London, July 13, 2013

CONCLUSION

In 2006 the Kentucky Nurses Association (KNA) published *Professional Nursing in Kentucky: Yesterday, Today, Tomorrow*, a historical overview of nursing in the state. Many of the nurses in this book echo the events recounted in the KNA book.

Professional Nursing in Kentucky traces the development of nursing to the early 1800s. "The records of nursing during this early period," the prologue explains, "are scanty, often conflicting, and difficult to discover. The first 'so-called nurses' in Kentucky and elsewhere in the Country were Roman Catholic Sisters. In times of epidemics they helped families care for their own when they fell victims to yellow fever, typhoid fever and cholera. The Sisters of Charity of Nazareth (SCN) were the first and only congregation of women religious to minister in the entire eastern half of Kentucky until 1859, when the Benedictine Sisters arrived in Covington."[1]

Nursing began to be established as a profession with the Crimean War in Europe (1853–1856) and the Civil War in the United States (1861–1865). "President Lincoln issued an appeal to religious orders for nurses. In Kentucky, Brigadier-General Robert Anderson and Bishop Martin J. Spalding requested volunteers from the Sisters of Charity of Nazareth and [also] the Dominican Sisters of St. Catherine. . . . The U. S. Sanitary Commission paid female nurses. The sisters and other church women volunteered by the hundreds in Kentucky to care for the Union and Confederate casualties of battles throughout the Commonwealth. Emergency hospitals were set up in school buildings (closed by war), factories, warehouses and even court houses."[2]

Professional nurse training programs followed, although "Kentucky did not begin to train women until more than two decades" after the Civil War. "Nationally, there were thirty-five schools of nursing by 1875, fifteen more by 1880, thirty-four more by 1885, and by this date, none in Kentucky. . . . Greatly influenced by the nursing school founded in London by Florence Nightingale at St. Thomas Hospital in 1860, several Nightingale patterned schools began in the U. S. . . . A school for nurses opened at the John N. Norton Memorial Infirmary in Louisville, 1886. Others followed, including those privately owned by physicians."[3]

The KNA, a professional organization for the entire state, was established in 1906, when

> a letter went out to nurse faculty and graduates of Kentucky training schools for nurses and nurses elsewhere, from the Nurses Alumna, Norton Infirmary (founded 1905) and the Jefferson County Nurses Club (founded 1896). The letter invited them to a meeting in Louisville November 28 and 29. . . . Sixty-nine nurses accepted the invitation. Records do not identify them, nor the areas from which they came. Travel was usually limited to train. Cars were few and road conditions poor. . . . Presentations by bishops, doctors and club women welcomed the nurses and offered encouragement and support.[4]

By midcentury, as the Cold War developed, nurses were envisioned to have a key role in civil defense preparedness.

> At the beginning of the 1950s, National Security was at the top of the government agenda. . . . Nursing was declared a critical occupation, for nurses would be expected to give primary health care in disasters, which might well result from atomic, chemical or bacteriological warfare. Committees and programs attempted to prepare nurses for such eventualities. The National Security Civil Defense Board made arrangements to provide regional courses of instruction, "The Nursing Aspects of Atomic Warfare," and they called on the state governors for assistance. Governor Wetherby appointed Margaret East, RN Director, Division of Public Health Nursing, State Department of Health to act as coordinator of civil defense.[5]

By the twenty-first century, the nursing profession had seen dramatic transformations, but the fundamental role of nurses remained unchanged in many ways. "As nurses face the unresolved problems of the last several decades," *Professional Nursing in Kentucky* explains, "they continue to be challenged by an ailing health care system that has changed little as it provides a high quality of service to a few. The

United States remains the only industrialized country in the world that does not provide health care to its populace. The underpinning of the nursing profession is caring as depicted in the American Nurses Association (ANA) *Code of Ethics.* Nurses care for patients, families or for anyone in need. Understandably then, a nurse feels pressured by the inherent ethical dilemma presented when men, women, and children are under-cared-for and under-insured."[6]

My personal contacts with nurses demonstrated how their services have undergone significant changes since the early twentieth century, as has the social and economic well-being of Kentuckians. Numerous stories in this book reflect the changes in nursing methods and in the attitudes of nurses since the days of walking, riding horses, and driving jeeps to reach persons in critical need.

The stories herein relate the histories and experiences of individual nurses, but they also describe traditional accounts recounted to them by patients or other nurses. The bountiful stories in this book describe what life, times, medications, and medical services were all about in early times and today. Nurses also expressed the importance of family and community wellness across the years.

My central purpose with this book is to provide personal memories of nurses, who willingly shared their feelings about the importance of nurses and doctors in the minds and hearts of people throughout the Commonwealth of Kentucky. The descriptions of crucial, dedicated services provided by these nurse-storytellers are essential for informing future nurses, doctors, and hospital laborers what their predecessors did to support patients' lives and health.

Notes

1. Marge Glaser and Maggie Miller, eds., *Professional Nursing in Kentucky: Yesterday, Today, Tomorrow* (Louisville: Kentucky Nurses Association, 2006), 9.
2. Ibid., 10–11.
3. Ibid.
4. Ibid., 17.
5. Ibid., 45.
6. Ibid., 81.

BIOGRAPHIES OF STORYTELLERS

EVELYN PEARL ANDERSON provided the following biographical sketch: "Growing up on a Fleming County, Kentucky, farm, I had only one dream and that was to be a nurse. However, my development as a potential artist was already beginning. I was influenced by the colors of nature that surrounded me on the farm and by working with my mother on dress design and sewing projects. When I reached high school I found myself as the one schoolmate called on to design posters for events. I still didn't think of myself as an artist. I fulfilled my dream and became an RN in 1961. A nursing career, marriage to my husband, Carlos, and raising a family of three kids kept me busy.

"When I returned to school at Campbellsville College I found myself wondering about art, Could I do it? Well, I majored in social work but minored in art. For a short time after graduating from Campbellsville College in 1977, I worked in acrylics and oils. I enjoyed some recognition but many other interests and responsibilities relative to church, family, completing an MSW [master of social work] degree with a gerontology concentration, [and a] career in nursing and health care management and teaching took over. Consequently I laid my paintbrushes aside for thirty years.

"After a serious illness that ended my full-time nursing career, I began writing prose and poetry, which led to my first published book, *Journey with the Wind* (2003). Then in 2009 a new dream took hold of me since I was a watercolor artist. I registered in a watercolor workshop, studied books and CDs, and got a bit of private instruction. Watercolor painting began to flow from me, along with poems and short stories. Thus *Pearl's Poetry of Watercolors* was born.

"I had written three additional books that were published by 2009. Two of them were memoirs, with titles *Daylite's A-Comin'* and *Knitted with Love*. The first was about me being a student nurse in a hospital school of nursing. The second is about a collection of handwritten entries made while on six short-term mission trips to southwestern Russia. I often refer to this as the book of my heart. *Patterns of Grace* was the last book published. It is a book that contains poetry of aging, which could be seen as a book of my life's work.

"I delight in capturing through written word or paint a bit of the beauty that God surrounds us with every day, whether it is a flower, a sunset, water falling, or an open field with grazing cattle. I truly feel it is a blessing to learn one's gift after seventy years of age.

"My husband, Carlos, and I live in London, Laurel County. We enjoy our three children and five grandchildren, two in London and three in Jakarta, Indonesia."

TERESA FRYMAN BELL stated, "I started nursing when I was nineteen and went to Appalachian School of Nursing, which is now known as Central Kentucky Bluegrass Tech College, which is located in Lexington. I am originally from a little Harrison County town called Berry, located fifty or seventy miles north of Lexington. I have four other siblings, but I was the only one to go to college.

"I recently graduated from Everest University online with an associate's degree in medical billing and coding. I worked full-time and maintained a 3.86 [grade point] average. I did this to show my children that regardless of our age we can do anything we put our minds to.

"My father's name was Marvin Fryman and my mother's name was Geneva Sue Fryman. My father had a full scholarship to play basketball when he graduated from high school but his father refused to let him go because he was needed on the farm. My father decided that he would never deny any of his children to go to college. We were very poor while growing up, but at the time we didn't know that because we had a lot of love in our home and our parents taught us values that I have taught my children.

"I started working to pay for my own gas to and from school, worked as a nurse's aide, and then babysat while going to nursing school. If we wanted something we had to work for it because things are just not given to you. I wish my parents were both here with me today to see all I have done in my life. I have four children, Brandon Miller, who graduated in 2005; Aaron Miller graduated in 2007; Kacee Miller graduated in 2011; and Morgan Miller is in high school as a freshman.

"I worked second shift in a hospital for a long time."

MARY LEWIS BIGGERSTAFF, a resident of Berea at the time she was interviewed, was born in Hyden in 1899. She tells of her pioneer background and also mentions some early residents of the area before the Frontier Nursing Service was established. She was present at the first organizational meeting of the FNS at the courthouse in Hyden in 1925.

Her father introduced Mary Breckinridge to many people in Leslie County. She also talks about black families and a black school in Hyden. She recalls the family histories of many Leslie County residents and gives the names and backgrounds of early doctors in the community, a grandmother who practiced public health, and also a number of early pharmacists.

Biggerstaff's recollection of buildings in Hyden is extremely specific. She relates her personal acquaintance with Mary Breckinridge at length. She also provides some details of the Deaton-Callahan feud, among other local happenings.

HELEN EDITH BROWNE stated, "I was born in a rural area of eastern England in the county of Suffolk, in a small village called Brushbrook. It had a population of probably 250. I grew up in the country and went to a private girls' school. Well, we had a governess to start with. I was the second child in the family and my brother, who was a year older than I was, [was] the one from whom I started to learn the alphabet. Until the age of ten we were taught by this governess, and then while living with my grandmother I went to day school in Ipswich, which is still in Suffolk. . . . After I finished high school . . . I wanted to be a nurse.

"My father didn't want me to become a nurse because he just thought it was not for me. I think my mother was seriously ill after my sister was born and we had nurses in the house for a long, long time. . . . So this introduced me to a lot of nurses and I wanted to become a nurse. However, my father said no, and he thought that maybe a secretarial career was better for me. He took me to several bank managers whom he knew . . . and they all said yes, but I finally decided that [banking] was not for me. . . . I went to London hospitals and was accepted. Finally my father had to give permission after my mother helped to persuade him this is what I wanted to do. So in 1930 I went to London and entered Bartholomew's Hospital School of Nursing for a three-year course. . . . You had to learn to work with doctors and in those days nursing medicine collaborated very closely in the care of patients.

"Back then most nurses in England, especially from the Big Five [hospitals] in London, went on to do midwifery. So after my year as a staff nurse and I was free to go, I decided to do midwifery, then got my midwifery certificate in 1935."

JANA BUCKLES of Lawrenceburg provided the following biographical information: "I have been a registered nurse for twenty-nine years and have seen all sorts of action during this time. I am board certified and have a double master's degree and a BSN. I was also a vet technician back when they were not popular. I am married to a wonderful man, Keith, and we have three dogs, all adopted. I have worked all areas except oncology and in the cath[eterization] lab in the hospital setting. I have been a staff nurse and worked my way up the food chain to the CNO [chief nursing officer] position.

"I am not a house supervisor in a one-hundred-bed hospital. I prefer smaller hospitals over large ones since it is a more intimate setting and one can have autonomy while working."

DANA BURNAM stated, "I was born in Bowling Green, June 28, 1976, but spent some time growing up in Russellville, starting in the sixth grade. I have been married to my husband, Ryan, for nine years. We have two daughters. The oldest is sixteen months and the youngest is five and one-half months old. We currently live in Plano, Kentucky.

"I graduated from the Western Kentucky University's ASN nursing program in 2011. I have worked at a medical center for fourteen years, on a postpartum floor at the medical center, and [in] the emergency room at the medical center in Bowling Green."

JENNY BURTON was born August 25, 1944, in Bowling Green, then graduated from Chandlers Chapel High School, Logan County, in 1962. As a little child she had the desire to become a nurse but really didn't know why. In 1973 she attended the Glasgow School for Practical Nurses. For one year she worked at a hospital in Annapolis, Maryland, then returned to Bowling Green in 1975, where she worked at Greenview Hospital until her retirement in 1999. She began working there again in 2003 and continues to work with a group called Industry and Wellness.

RUTH A. BUZZARD has been married to the same man for fifty-six years and has two children and four grandchildren. She was employed as a registered nurse for forty years, twenty of which were spent in nursing service and twenty in nursing education. She received a BSN from Murray State University and an MSN (master of science in nursing) from the University of Evansville. She retired from the University of Kentucky Community College System, Hopkinsville Community College, and currently resides in Dawson Springs, Hopkins County.

DOROTHY CALDWELL first went to the FNS as a courier in 1938. She discusses her experiences in taking care of the horses at Wendover and going on rounds with such persons as Betty Lester. During the interview she talks about Betty Lester's changing role as an FNS administrator. Caldwell explains what the FNS meant to couriers and expresses her feelings about the job she performed. She also talks extensively about Mary Breckinridge, her administration of the FNS, and her life at Wendover.

After Caldwell left the FNS she worked at Cincinnati General Hospital and was active in the Cincinnati FNS Committee.

(The foregoing was provided by Caldwell's interviewer, Marion Barrett.)

REBECCA COLLINS attended Western Kentucky University School of Nursing and received an associate's degree in the nursing program in 1985. Subsequently she received her bachelor's degree from Western Kentucky University in 1990. She served as learning resource coordinator at Western Kentucky, and worked as a nurse in the Critical Care Unit at Greenview Hospital, 1985–2007.

MICHELE DEGOTT provided valuable thoughts and insights in an account in chapter 9. Biographical information is not available.

JEAN FEE began working for the Frontier Nursing Service during the fall of 1958, after responding to an ad in the *American Journal of Nursing*. After her arrival in Hyden, she explains, she "worked the next five or six months in the hospital in the general side, spent the next six months in the school of midwifery, graduating from there during the fall [of] 1959. Then I worked during the winter [of] 1959 through spring of 1961 in various districts. I received my permanent district in the spring of 1960 and that was the first of the districts that Mrs. Breckinridge had organized outside of her home in Wendover."

TERESA M. "TERRY" FOODY received a BS in nursing from Niagara University New York and a master's degree in nursing from the University of Kentucky. She is also a certified clinical research coordinator through the Association of Clinical Research Professionals. Her experiences include community nursing in New York State, school health nursing in Kentucky, teaching nursing students at Kentucky State University, and coordinating research trials at the University of Kentucky. She has a speaking and consulting business on healthy living in the areas of nutrition, fitness, and stress hardiness. She has extensively researched and presented on the cholera epidemics of the nineteenth century, citing implications for our global health today.

She is a speaker for the Kentucky Humanities Council and has written a book about the 1833 cholera epidemic in central Kentucky that includes three heroes: the Pie-Seller, the Drunk, and the Society Matron.

She can be found online at www.TerryFoody.com.

CAROLYN BOOTH GREGORY, born July 21, 1925, learned about the Frontier Nursing Service while a student at Bates College in Lewiston, Maine. Following her graduation in the late 1940s she volunteered to work as Christmas secretary at the FNS and organized the donation of gifts for local children. In her interview she discusses Christmas at the FNS and the family atmosphere throughout the organization. For the remainder of the year she performed clerical tasks and served as a part-time courier.

The FNS impressed her as a community of self-sufficient women, and she recounts a number of experiences during the transition from horses to jeeps. She also comments about visits with local people and recalls being present at several births.

(Gregory provided the foregoing comments to interviewer Linda Green.)

DR. MARY Q. HAWKES of Newton, Massachusetts, worked in Leslie County with a group at the Stinnett Settlement School while in college and began work with the FNS in 1948 in social services. She talks about the differences between training in social work and actually working in a place where no agencies exist to assist people in need. Hawkes discusses the "Kentucky Mountain Male Syndrome," in which men raised in the mountains to do seasonal work could not adjust to working by a time clock. Once they began to have to meet a school bus, children made the transition and became accustomed to time constraints.

Hawkins also remarks on the impact of television on mountain localities. She explains her role as liaison between the FNS and the Kentucky Crippled Children Commission and talks about some child welfare cases. She discusses the lives of the nurses at Wendover and their association with Mary Breckinridge. She goes on to comment on local living conditions and the influence of various technological changes in the mid-1960s.

(Hawkins provided the foregoing comments to interviewer Dale Deaton.)

MARTHA LAINE ULM HILL stated, "I was born in Cairo, Georgia, and lived with my parents in Thomasville, Georgia, until I was ten years old, when my father moved us to North Carolina, where he opened his automobile mechanic business. I lived in North Carolina until I went away to college after graduating from high school in 1962. I attended Berea College and received my bachelor's in nursing from there, then worked for a year in Louisville at Methodist Evangelical Hospital. I then became engaged to my husband and we married; then I worked at Berea Hospital for a while and then came to Elizabethtown in 1968, where I became an instructor of nursing at Elizabethtown Community College. I then went to the University of Kentucky and received my master's degree in nursing. The remaining portion of my nursing career was spent at Elizabethtown Community College, at which I became chairman of the nursing degree program and remained there from 1984 until my retirement in 1997.

"Since then I have done some consulting events for nursing education and have truly enjoyed retirement after that."

In addition to her nursing and teaching services across the years, Hill also served as a consultant, hospital staff member, program evaluator, and chairperson, president, and vice president on nominating committees. She also provided lecture presentations to various groups in Idaho, Illinois, Indiana, Kentucky, Massachusetts, New Mexico, and Texas.

FREDERICKA HOLDSHIP first came to the Frontier Nursing Service in 1937 after having heard Mary Breckinridge speak at a meeting. She recalls her first trip to Wendover by bus and horseback and also goes into detail concerning the different FNS centers and the nurses associated with them. Holdship tells of Breckinridge's efforts to obtain horses during World War II and various ways in which problems were managed at Wendover. She talks about the routine of the nurses and the difficulty of getting away for any time off and describes the raising of children and the life of the local people.

She also conducted research on children's aptitude or excellence. She became chairperson of the Pittsburgh Committee in 1969 and later was appointed to the FNS Board of Governors.

GERTRUDE ISAACS, who has her doctorate in nursing, was codirector of the Family Nurse Practitioner Program at the Frontier School of Midwifery and Family Nursing with Dr. W. B. Rogers Beasley in 1971, and then she was named education director of the school. In 1977 she became a consultant to the school.

In her interview, Isaacs speaks of her acquaintance with Mary Breckinridge and of what the FNS meant to the local people. She discusses Breckinridge's philosophy of preventive care and teaching people to care for themselves. She comments on the change in atmosphere in FNS relations with local residents after the nurses stopped visiting in the homes. She believes that part of what Breckinridge created has been lost through overregulation by federal and state governments and by Medicare and Medicaid.

Isaacs also discusses the controversy over physician support of nurse midwives and the increasing demand for home deliveries. Besides giving statistics, Isaacs clarifies a number of terms, differentiating between primary medical care and primary health care. She also discusses social relations within the mountain family and the position of children.

(Isaacs's interviewer, Dale Deaton, provided the foregoing comments based on interviews conducted in 1978 and 1980.)

THERESA SUE MILBURN KING was born in Danville, Kentucky, December 6, 1946, as the only daughter of William Isaac "Tobe" Milburn and Theresa Holtzclaw Milburn. King was a 1963 graduate of Danville High School, a 1967 graduate of Vanderbilt University School of Nursing, and 1977 graduate of the University of Kentucky. She was a registered nurse for over forty years. Her nursing practice encompassed hospital nursing, vocational nursing education, Medicaid nurse aide instruction, first aid nursing with Rupp Arena and the University of Kentucky, and independent contracting of insurance physicals.

King was appointed to the Kentucky Board of Nursing in 1990 and served through 1994. She was active in the Kentucky Nurses Association, District 9 KNA, and the American Nurses Association. In recognition of her service she was awarded lifetime membership in 1999. In 2005 King was selected as Examiner of the Year by Portamedic/ Hooper Holmes for the eastern portion of the United States. She was commissioned as a Kentucky Colonel and is a member of Sigma Theta Tau and several alumni organizations.

She currently resides in Boyle County, Kentucky. Her present interests include Kentucky history and genealogy, along with various crafts (tatting, quilting, basketry, and nurturing her yard).

MARY LANSING was a friend of Mary Breckinridge, as was Lansing's mother, Elizabeth Lansing. The latter visited Wendover in 1946 to conduct research for a book about the FNS entitled *Rider on the Mountains*, which was published the following year.

Mary Lansing served as a courier during the summer of 1968. She recalls assisting nurse-midwives with medical treatment and helping to transport children from the area to a hospital in Cincinnati. Lansing, who was working in a congressional office at the time of the interview [no stories included], believes that the Appalachian region is still not sufficiently understood by government leaders and outsiders in general.

(Lansing's interviewer, Anne Campbell Ritchie, provided the foregoing comments.)

GEORGIA LEDFORD has family members who have served on the Clay County Committee of the Frontier Nursing Service and have worked for this organization in various capacities.

Ledford recalls her association with Mary Breckinridge and details the activities of the nurse-midwives by commenting on their effectiveness and the impact of the Frontier Nursing Service in the local area. Ledford also includes a description of handmade furniture.

(Ledford's interviewer, Carol Crowe-Carraco, provided the foregoing comments.)

MOLLY LEE came to the Frontier Nursing Service from England as a nurse-midwife, having had experience in England, Scotland, and Canada. Part of her district nursing experience as a Queen's Nurse had been learning to do without the usual supplies and to improvise in people's homes. Lee describes her midwifery course in England in detail and compares it to the curriculum in the United States, the latter being more comprehensive.

She began work with the FNS in 1955, serving at Beech Fork and later at Confluence. Having left the FNS for a period of time, Lee returned in 1958 to teach at the hospital. She also performed most of the home deliveries in the Hyden area.

Lee discusses Mary Breckinridge, in particular as a speaker at a fund-raising dinner. She also explains that the amended Kentucky law, as of the time of the interview, prevented nurse-midwives from being paid for deliveries if a doctor was not present, a circumstance that negated their purpose, and that outside of Kentucky midwives were recognized and paid.

Lee also discusses the birth control pill developed by Dr. John

Rook and its reception in the FNS area. She goes on to detail the current operation of the FNS and the teaching program. Lee also specifies some innovative procedures needed in delivery and comments on midwifery examinations.

(Lee provided the foregoing comments to interviewer Carol Crowe-Carraco.)

BETTY LESTER received her nurse training in London, England, beginning in 1939. She recalls numerous tales about midwives, often referred to as family nurses, as part of her personal experience in the Frontier Nursing Service in England. Thanks to FNS founder Mary Breckinridge, Lester came to the Frontier Nursing Service in Hyden, Kentucky, upon returning from England in July 1928. Both of Lester's parents died before she started nursing.

She was a resident of Hyden when Jonathan Freid interviewed her in 1978. According to Freid, during the interview "Lester mentions the high maternal mortality rate in Leslie County before the FNS arrived. . . . She talks about the building on Wendover and the small hospital. Lester goes into details of how services were set up and the nurses established in district centers. . . . She also described the Frontier Graduate School of Midwifery, begun during World War II."

(The foregoing information was gathered from Lester's interview and from comments by interviewer Jonathan Freid.)

AGNES LEWIS was hired by Mary Breckinridge in 1930, when Lewis was about thirty, to work in the FNS records department. Lewis describes an eventful trip to Wendover, in the course of which she had to look after two children returning from the hospital in Cincinnati. When Lewis arrived at Wendover, many people were leaving; thus she was assuming great and unfamiliar responsibilities. Lewis describes Mary Breckinridge and recounts some of their conversations. She also refers to Breckinridge's father, who conducted various small projects on the grounds and lived at Wendover until his death in 1932.

Lewis goes on to discuss the drought and the Great Depression, which occurred in succession. The Red Cross came in at Breckinridge's request and determined allotments to be given to local families. Lewis also tells of Breckinridge's fall from a new horse and describes the effects of the accident. Besides her mention of many local people who assisted the FNS, Lewis identifies a number of the FNS staff.

Lewis handled the bills owed by the FNS during the 1930s and

1940s and indicates the difficulties faced by the organization during the period, including a flu epidemic and the necessity of cutting nurses' salaries. Lewis comments at length on the character of the mountain people. She also tells of two near-lawsuits and how they were avoided. In addition, Lewis explains the philosophy behind the regulations observed by the FNS nurses.

(Lewis's interviewer, Dale Deaton, provided the foregoing comments.)

ELSIE MAIER said, "I went to nursing school in New York City thanks to a diploma program through the City of New York Hospitals–Queens Hospital School of Nursing, and that was a three-year program. After that I went to Barrington College for two years and got my BA degree. Right away after that, in 1962, I came to Frontier Nursing Service and took the six-month midwifery course and became a certified nurse-midwife.

"I found out about FNS through an FNS graduate who was working in Guatemala. That was between my two years in college. I was impressed when I met the FNS grad. I went to Vanderbilt University in 1973 to get my master's degree in family nursing.

"I worked at FNS from 1962 to 1972, then went on leave of absence from 1972 to 1974. During that time I was in Africa; then I came back for a couple of weeks and then went on to college."

MARILYN KAYE MONTELL, born 1954, is a Monroe County native, daughter of Charles and Elizabeth (Bowman) Montell. Upon completion of nurse training with the American Diabetic Association (ADA) at Midway College School of Nursing in 1976, she worked a few years in an emergency room in Louisville. Most recently, she has worked for twelve years in the cardiac cath lab as a traveling nurse employed by the Medsource company, based in Florida. Due to the importance of her job with Medsource, she has served at numerous hospitals located in Maine, New Hampshire, California, Montana, Washington state, Colorado, Georgia, Kentucky, Tennessee, Indiana, Wisconsin, Vermont, Nebraska, Kansas, Illinois, Iowa, Florida, and Louisiana.

In her words, "I went into nursing because Grandma [Montell] told me I should, and I always listened to her advice because she was usually right."

CHESA MONTGOMERY graduated from Western Kentucky University School of Nursing, served as a nurse at the Medical Center, Bowling

Green, then worked in the emergency room at Greenview Regional Hospital, also in Bowling Green. All total, she served as a nurse for twenty years and still resides in Bowling Green.

CARRIE M. PARKER offers information about her mother, who was born in Leslie County in 1900, then later went to a nursing school in Philadelphia. She returned to Leslie County as a public health nurse before Mary Breckinridge founded the Frontier Nursing Service and became acquainted with Ms. Breckinridge while working at the original hospital in Hyden, Kentucky.

Parker herself was born in 1945 and resided during the 1950s with her parents in Laurel County, where she attended school through eighth grade, then completed high school in Leslie County. She later went to the University of Kentucky and Rawlings College in Virginia.

Parker became a junior courier for the FNS with Carlyle Carter, a cousin of Mary Breckinridge. Parker recalls her family becoming severely affected by union strife because of her father's involvement in the coal industry. She served as a courier in 1966, after the death of Mary Breckinridge, and comments on the change in atmosphere upon her return to the FNS.

Eventually Parker joined the city committee in Washington, D.C., She reflects on both mountain and outside societies from the perspective of one who has been a part of each.

(The bulk of the foregoing comments were provided by Parker to interviewer Dale Deaton.)

JOYCE PARRISH, native of Dunmor, Muhlenberg County, received nurse training at the University of Louisville. Then, beginning about 1960, she worked various types of jobs at Logan Memorial Hospital, Russellville, where she remained for more than fifty years.

MARY PENTON attended the FNS Graduate School of Midwifery from 1957 to 1958 after working for six months in general nursing. The FNS paid her tuition in exchange for her agreement to stay for at least a year and a half. Penton eventually stayed for eight and a half years. She worked for five years at the Flat Creek Center, doing home health work as well as nursing and midwifery. She discusses the operation of the center and changes in FNS policies across the years. Penton also comments on area trends in regard to birth control and family planning. Additional topics are the different drugs used for pain during delivery events and the introduction of bottle feeding in the Frontier Nursing Service area. She left in 1965.

(Penton's interviewer, Dale Deaton, provided the foregoing comments.)

NANCY N. PORTER graduated from Harper Hospital, Birmingham, Michigan, in 1946 and then went to the FNS as a nurse in 1947. She recalls Christmas in Wendover, Leslie County, and the preparation of clothing to be given away. Porter served in the hospital clinic and describes her work as well as the hospital facilities at that time.

Porter's contact with Wendover was minimal during this period, since she had no midwifery training and did not go out on local visits. She talks a bit about hospital facilities and obstetrical care in Detroit, and discusses the Detroit Committee of the FNS. She also comments on the FNS's *Quarterly Bulletin.*

(Porter's interviewer, Dale Deaton, provided the foregoing comments.)

GRACE REEDER first learned of the Frontier Nursing Service when she heard Mary Breckinridge speak at a meeting in Cincinnati. She asked Breckinridge for permission to join the FNS, received permission, and came to Hyden in 1939. After volunteering for a month as a staff nurse in the hospital in Hyden, Reeder came back in 1941 as a member of the regular staff and became chief nurse in the outpatient department. She later graduated from the FNS Graduate School of Midwifery and remained for three years as a district nurse.

Reeder tells of her work with the local people to avoid moonshine stills on her rounds and of helping children go to Berea College's Foundation School. Throughout her interview she discusses local ideas about property and attitudes toward the FNS nurses throughout the duration of her experience.

(Reeder's interviewer, Carol Crowe-Carraco, provided the foregoing comments.)

BOBBI DAWN RIGHTMYER says, "I was born in historic Harrodsburg, Kentucky. I have lived here all my life. When I was seventeen years old I graduated from Mercer County High School, 1980, in the number-four position of 276 students, and had been married for six months. Two years later my first daughter was born, and then my second daughter followed eighteen months later. As [with] most marriages of teenagers,

I went through a nasty divorce at the age of twenty-three and was left as a single mother with two small children." She recounts her experience in nursing school in chapter 7.

Rightmyer continued, "I realize most nursing teachers recommend that you get a year's experience working medical-surgical nursing but I wanted to work labor and delivery and was lucky enough to be able to get a job in my field of interest. For the next fifteen years I worked night shift in the birthing center at Ephraim McDowell Regional Medical Center in Danville. Although I liked my job, I had tried to get on day shift almost from the beginning. Working night shift was hard when I was newly married and raising two growing daughters, plus the new addition to our family, another daughter (Christine Nicole).

"In 2001 I decided to take a day shift job working at my local hospital, the James B. Haggin Memorial Hospital. Going from nights to days was a harder adjustment than I had planned, but it worked much better with my family. The problem was I realized I did not like working with medical-surgical patients. I was working day shift but not at a job I enjoyed. Six months later I took another leap of faith and became assessment coordinator in the Extended Care Unit of the same hospital.

"I know the old saying 'never say never' is a true one because I always said I never wanted to work in a nursing home, but there I was working in a nursing home. I found out almost immediately that working with the elderly was wonderful and fulfilling.

"My sister, Amy (Carter) Sallee, was in nursing school when she died of a heart attack at age thirty-nine. I had trouble going back to work [after that] because I found no joy in nursing. I realized I had fulfilled my goal, which was 'go to nursing school and raise my children.' It was 2005 and my children were raised by then, and I knew this was time for my life to take another turn. I have been retired from nursing for over seven years, and although there are aspects of the career I miss, I am enjoying this new phase in my life."

(Rightmyer provided the foregoing comments to the author, Lynwood Montell.)

DR. KAY T. ROBERTS (legal name Katherine Thompson Long Roberts) was born November 11, 1940, in Morganfield, Union County, to William Jones "Shorty" Long and Emma Catherine (Thompson) Long. Her paternal grandparents were the wealthy William Jones Long, known as "B," and Lily Henry (Fellows) Long, both of whom were from eastern Kentucky. Her grandparents moved to Morganfield during the Civil War and ran a cleaning and pressing shop that attracted Camp Breckinridge soldiers; upon retirement they purchased a farm, where her grandfather sold food and livestock, thus prompting Kay to love farmland and farming. Kay's maternal grandparents were Edward Royce Thompson and Helen Calita (Gough) Thompson.

After twelve years of schooling at St. Vincent Academy, Kay graduated from high school in 1958 in a class of twenty-two students. At almost age eighteen, Kay married John C. Wright III, age twenty-five, who later served as a doctor and was Kay's life partner for twenty-two years. After marriage, she worked as a lab assistant at Morganfield Hospital and about one year later became a nursing assistant. Later Kay and her husband moved to Henderson, where their two sons, Joseph and Daniel, were born, and where she worked as a lab/office assistant for an internal medicine physician.

After Henderson Community College opened in the 1960s, Kay enrolled in one class in 1965 but went on to graduate in 1967 with an extremely high GPA. She later attended the University of Evansville, from which she graduated in 1970 with a BSN degree. She began work as a nursing administrator at the local hospital and also began teaching at the University of Louisville. She completed a master's degree in the science of nursing in 1976 and received a doctoral degree in higher education administration from Indiana University in 1983. She accepted a faculty position at the University of Louisville in 1986 and was recruited as a gerontological nurse.

Across the years, Dr. Roberts has served in various positions and, along with teaching, has helped develop several dynamic centers designed to serve patient needs.

(Roberts provided the foregoing information to the author, Lynwood Montell.)

KAREN SLABAUGH received an associate's degree in nursing from Mott Community College in Flint, Michigan, during the early 1960s, then learned about the Frontier Nursing Service while serving as a nurse in Costa Rica and subsequently went through FNS family nurse and midwifery training. She gives details of the curriculum and explains how the two programs overlapped. She also describes the range of a midwife's skills and duties.

Slabaugh sees nursing experience with the FNS as providing an effective laboratory for the success of persons like herself who wish to serve in other isolated rural locations throughout the world.

(Slabaugh's interviewer, Dale Deaton, provided the foregoing comments.)

PATRICIA A. SLATER, a current resident of Petersburg, Boone County, was born in Covington and grew up in Erlanger, Kenton County. She attended Lloyd Memorial High School and St. Elizabeth School of Nursing, from which she graduated in 1960. She married in 1964, moved to Massachusetts, where she lived for eighteen months, and then moved back to Cincinnati, where her husband was completing his PhD at the University of Cincinnati. They then returned to Massachusetts, where they resided for two years while her husband was working in a postdoc position at MIT. They later returned to Cincinnati, where her husband taught in the Aerospace Engineering Department at the university and they became parents of four children.

From 1957 to 1999 Patricia worked in nursing positions, primarily as a staff nurse at hospitals in Covington; Louisville; Waltham, Massachusetts; and Lawrenceburg, Indiana. During the 1960–1961 school year she served as a women's residence health nurse at Eastern Kentucky State Teachers College in Richmond. In 1978 she completed a BA degree in psychology. In 1986 she completed the BSN from Northern Kentucky University, and in 1988 the MSN from the University of Cincinnati. She retired from a faculty position at the College of Mount St. Joseph on the Ohio in 1998. In 1999 she became a volunteer executive director of United Ministries, a special service agency in Erlanger, utilizing the skills developed throughout her nursing career.

Patricia stays very active in gardening, sewing, knitting, church activities, and travel. Her volunteer work continues, as she sews caps for the American Cancer Society for women undergoing chemotherapy and occasionally does workshops for other volunteers at United Ministries.

CLARA FAY SMITH was born in Blackey, Kentucky, and graduated from Letcher County High School. She studied nursing at Berea College, even though her family thought she should major in something worthwhile that she could teach—such as English. Upon graduating in 1965, she accepted a nursing position at the William Booth Memorial Hospital in Covington, Kentucky. Soon after, she was promoted to assistant head nurse on a medical-surgical floor. In 1971 she accepted a public health nursing position at the Family Planning Clinic in Covington, Kentucky, where she served as both a clinic nurse and a family life nurse educator for eighteen years. In 1989 she became the district school nurse for the Erlanger-Elsmere Board of Education, where she worked for ten years before retiring. She remains active in retirement, volunteering as a reading coach in the one-to-one literacy program at Arnett Elementary School and as a tutor of elementary school children. She plays the dulcimer for her students in music class and serves on the advisory councils of both the Family Resource Center and the Youth Service Center of the Erlanger-Elsmere School District.

JANET SMITH, a resident of Irvine, has worked at Marcum and Wallace Memorial Hospital, especially in the emergency room, for several years.

LYDIA THOMPSON did her nurse training in Leeds and her midwifery in Glasgow, Scotland. She was about thirty years old at the time she came to America and heard about the Frontier Nursing Service in eastern Kentucky. She was with the FNS from July 1947 until the summer of 1952. She heard about the FNS from a friend of her sister and was truly interested in horses and riding. In her words, "I thought it'd be rather nice to do my district nursing on horseback. I wrote to the Frontier Nursing Service and told them I was interested. That was just after the war, so Mrs. Breckinridge wrote back and sent a lot of information and said I could come as soon as I liked. It took me about a year to get a visa. I paid my own way to get here but was refunded when I got here."

She left Liverpool en route to America and arrived in New York in about ten days. She was met by the Red Cross in New York, then came to Kentucky via train to Lexington. From there she rode a bus to Hazard, then was transported on a jeep or a bus to Hyden, where she was met by Betty Lester, who took her up to the hospital during the middle of July, when it was very hot. In Thompson's words, "I was absolutely baked! I hadn't been there long until Betty Brown came in with a rattle she'd got from a rattlesnake, so I nearly turned around and went home! The heat and humidity were so bad I found it difficult to cope with.

"I was taken to Wendover the next day and met Mrs. Mary Breckinridge.

"The Frontier Nursing Service had an important mission when I was there in the 1950s. They did good work, but really this district nursing service was the same as what is being done here now and for ages. It's a wonderful tradition over here [in eastern Kentucky].

"I left the Frontier Nursing Service after I thought I had been there long enough; besides, I wanted to see more of America. I went out to New Mexico and worked with a doctor who had been in the Frontier

Nursing Service and also with another midwife, called Peggy Brown. We did midwifery and district nursing there in New Mexico, mainly with Spanish[-speaking] people.

"I left New Mexico and went to Seattle, Washington, where I worked in a hospital there that delivered babies. I guess I had worked long enough, but I did move on to Canada and worked there for two years, stopped working, then came back to Kentucky in 1956. My experiences were very rewarding because I learned about people and how important that is in this life."

(Thompson provided the foregoing comments to her interviewer, Carol Crowe-Carraco.)

JEAN TOLK did her nursing training in Grand Rapids, Michigan. Before the advent of the Frontier Nursing Service, she was familiar with the lack of medical facilities in Leslie County, Kentucky. The Louisville Public Health Department sent her as a public health nurse to provide medical assistance to local residents in the absence of two itinerant doctors. During her interview by Dale Deaton, Tolk talked about the establishment of a small dispensary at Dryhill, Leslie County, where she provided vaccinations and minor medical treatment. She also described the town of Hyden during that period and talked about conditions in Leslie County during the Depression, when government relief provided unfamiliar foods such as grapefruit.

CHARLENE VAUGHT, a Kentucky native but current resident of Portland, Tennessee, initially worked in the OB Department at Hopkins County Hospital, Madisonville, Kentucky. She also worked at nursing homes as a nurse's aide, especially at the Gowan Nursing Home, Robinson, Illinois, and at Pleasant Acres Nursing Home, Altamont, Illinois.

LOUISE WEBB was born in Munster, Germany, in 1980, then attended Scarborough College in England, 1991–1998. She graduated from Bournemouth University, England, in 2005 with a BSN, then married and moved to Bowling Green, Kentucky, where she attended Western Kentucky University. She graduated in 2011 with an MSN degree and went on to become a family nurse practitioner at Sahetya Medical Institute, Bowling Green.

MARTHA WEBSTER, a resident of Appletree, Ohio, when she was interviewed in 1979, tells of her experience as a Frontier Nursing Service courier in 1938. She tells about riding horses along extremely crude roads and recalls the courtesy of the mountaineers and the camaraderie among the nurses. A current member of the Cleveland Committee, Webster has not had recent contact with the Frontier Nursing Service.

(Webster's interviewer, Dale Deaton, provided the bulk of the foregoing comments.)

JO ANN M. WEVER, resident of Springfield, served at first on a medical-surgical floor, then as a nurse in the pediatric intensive care unit at the University of Kentucky Medical Center, Lexington. She was the featured nurse for numerous patients.

JERI R. WHITE lives in Lexington. Biographical information is not available.

GEORGE W. WILLIAMS was born in Laurel County in 1942, graduated from Hazel Green High School, then attended Berea College and Sue Bennett Junior College. He later enrolled in the nursing program at George Mason University, Fairfax, Virginia. At age nineteen he married a sixteen-year-old girl, and they have been married fifty-one years. George served as an army officer during the Vietnam War. At age forty-five he received a BS degree in nursing, and for the next twenty-two years he worked in the field he truly loved, especially in the hospital emergency room. Williams retired on his sixty-sixth birthday, and he and his wife reside in London, Kentucky.

(Williams provided the foregoing information to the author, Lynwood Montell.)

ANNE WINSLOW was recruited by Marvin Breckinridge Patterson to operate an FNS office in New York City. Following her graduation from Vassar in 1930, Winslow spent the summer in Leslie County, Kentucky, learning about the Frontier Nursing Service along with the nurse-midwives at the hospital in Hyden, or at outpost centers. Winslow recounts various experiences from her visits to the homes of local people.

She ran the New York office for three years and was responsible for publicity, fund-raising, and cooperation with the New York Committee. She also described the extensive efforts of Mary Breckinridge, along with stories about moonshine whiskey makers, revenue officers, and dangerous events related to them.

(Winslow's interviewer, Anne Campbell Ritchie, provided the foregoing comments.)

Mary Wiss came to the Frontier Nursing Service as medical director in October 1965 after having been a Sister of Charity in India, and she remained with the FNS until June 1969. She indicates some of the difficulties she encountered at the FNS concerning personnel and equipment and contrasts those circumstances with her experience in India. Wiss believes that most of the persons seen at district clinics could as easily have come to the hospital, thus eliminating the difficulty and the expense of maintaining these centers.

She discusses the attitude of the American Medical Association toward midwives and gives her own perspective. Wiss asserts that the local people, being much more sophisticated than formerly, and many being college educated, could have been given a larger role in the operation of the FNS than they were performing in the late 1960s.

Wiss also discusses the incidence of various health problems and of malnutrition.

(Wiss's interviewer, Dale Deaton, provided the foregoing comments.)

Index of Stories by County, Other States, and Countries

Kentucky Counties

Letcher

Other States